THE MID-LIFE DIET FOR WOMEN

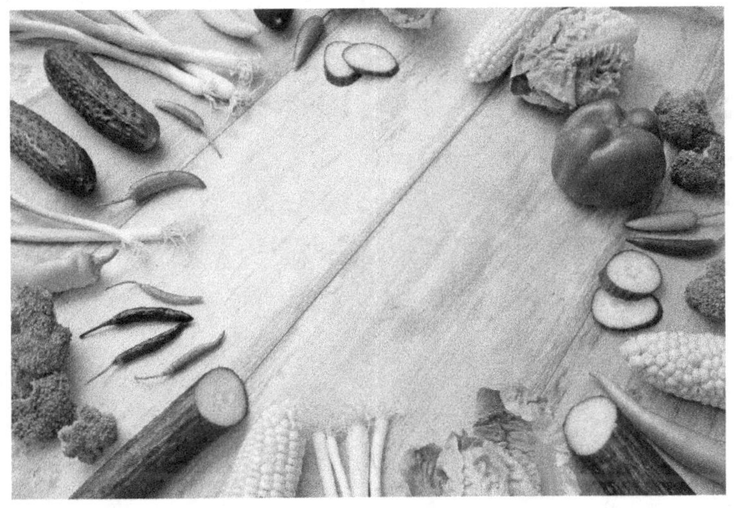

Evelyn T. Myers

<u>THE MID-LIFE DIET FOR WOMEN</u>

"Discover ways of living a fulfilling, healthy life in your Middle Ages through fasting intermittently, Anti-inflammatory Nutrition and Fat adapted dieting"

Legal Disclaimer

This book and its contents are not intended

to substitute any form of medical or

professional guidance; nor are they intended

to replace the need for independent medical,

financial, legal, or other professional advice

or services that may be required. This book's

content and information are offered solely for educational and entertaining reasons.

The content and information in this book were compiled from credible sources and are accurate to the best of the Author's knowledge, information, and belief. However, the Author cannot guarantee its authenticity or validity and, as a result, cannot be held liable for any errors or omissions. This book is also updated regularly as needed.

Before implementing any of the suggested cures, strategies, and/or information in this book, you should consult a professional (including but not limited to your doctor, attorney, financial adviser, or other such professional) if appropriate and/or necessary.

Table of contents

Introduction 7

Chapter 1 19

Midlife changes 19

Chapter 2 57

Taking control of your hormones 57

Chapter 3 85

Intermittent Fasting 85

Chapter 4 251

Anti-inflammatory Nutrition 251

Chapter 5 279

Fuel Refocus 279

Conclusions 307

Introduction

When a woman with polycystic ovarian syndrome (PCOS) came into my office for the first time, I had no idea what to do for her. She was dealing with weight gain in addition to many uncomfortable symptoms of the disease. Given my personal experience with conception issues, I was overjoyed when Dr. Stacy expressed interest in forming a collaboration between the fertility and nutrition departments at the large medical practice in Texas where I worked as a nutritionist and she as a fertility specialist. Stacy had provided me with medical attention, and we had grown close during my therapy. She was a big fan of the nutritionist in the practice. As a result, when she began to see women with PCOS, she turned to us for assistance. We were flattered as nutritionists, but we weren't certain that we could help these women at the time. I had no idea what this strange-sounding ailment was, let alone how diet and lifestyle could affect it. But Stacy was convinced that we would create an excellent team and, in the end, make a difference in the lives of these women. As I tried to cobble together some form of food therapy, she carefully explained PCOS to me and answered my queries.

I have my nutritionist team for collaboration. Steph, my biochemistry nutritionist colleague, likes nothing more than arguing the benefits of enzymes and chemical pathways. Next, I contacted New York nutritionist Margaret, who eagerly shared her knowledge of the illness with me. The key to figuring out how to manage PCOS nutritionally was discovering that insulin resistance is the most common cause of the disorder, which I was already familiar with. Two of my five siblings had type 1 diabetes as children, which is characterized by a deficiency of the pancreatic hormone insulin.

Insulin resistance, a disease characterized by inefficient use of this hormone, is the root cause of type 2 diabetes, which is the most frequent kind of diabetes in the United States. This early introduction to the realm of diabetes treatment piqued my curiosity about becoming a dietician. I began treating patients with PCOS using my expertise in how to manage insulin resistance. Initially, there were only a few patients, but the number has since climbed to several hundred. One thing was clear: the women with PCOS had many symptoms and complaints, and the majority of them felt mistreated by the medical system.

I found that many dietitians knew very little about this illness, and many of them began to seek my advice. I created a presentation on PCOS management for dietitians in my area; I repeatedly had the same feedback: "I know nothing about this" and "Oh my God, I think I have it!" This was not surprising given that women make up more than 97 percent of certified dietitians! As we began to meet more women with PCOS in our medical practice, the nutritionists and fertility and endocrinology department started organizing group support courses for women with PCOS, many of whom were overjoyed to find a safe space to discuss their health.

Many of these women shared the experience of knowing for years that something was wrong but never receiving much satisfaction or symptom relief from their doctors. We had young women, older women (who were just figuring out the diagnosis despite years of fertility treatments!), straight women, gay women, teenage girls, and their mothers, women trying to get pregnant, and women with no interest in children but a strong interest in avoiding diabetes. Despite some tough relationships, we kept the group going for a few years until the physicians left the practice (Stacy went to the Midwest) and the pressures of our employment as nutritionists forced us to leave.

Every year, millions of women around the world go through menopause, a universal feminine experience. Although some women breeze through the transition with little difficulty, three out of every four experience symptoms as a result of the huge variations in the female hormones estrogen and progesterone during this time, and one out of every four experiences severe symptoms. The most common symptoms are bothersome hot flashes, drenching night sweats, disrupted sleep, mood swings, vaginal dryness, sexuality concerns, and concerns about memory slippage, all of which can have an impact on a woman's most important relationships as well as her ability to function effectively at home and work.

After assisting women with various health conditions over the years in developing a diet and lifestyle that will help improve their overall well-being, I decided it would be beneficial to write a book for women in their mid-life; those in their perimenopause stages on their way to menopause. This book will help you get to know your body and teach you how to treat it like a loving friend by providing insight on menopause issues, the science behind how macronutrients support midlife health, sugar detoxing, hormonal balancing, long-term weight loss, and a healthy transition through perimenopause and menopause to postmenopause.

You will gain mental peace by learning how to establish new habits that bring you joy and improve your health, as well as work with your body to make you seem strong, slim, and attractive. This book is made up of three parts: They are essentially health-promoting acts that make the program work for you by forming excellent habits. All habits are formed by activities, learning, and repetition, resulting in the behavior being automatic. In other words, you do it instinctively. You will work on three acts at the same time to create excellent habits:

1. Intermittent fasting: This practice offers great benefits for women in terms of hormone balance, metabolism, and inflammation reduction. This is the most important component of the program for the majority of women. They said they felt better after learning how to fast intermittently.

2. Anti-inflammatory nutrition: Chronic inflammation, the root cause of many disorders, causes weight gain. However,

weight growth also causes inflammation, so the two feed off each other in a bizarre cycle. Women's inflammation worsens as we age and undergo menopausal hormone swings. A lot of the items we eat don't help either because they produce inflammation throughout the body.

However, this does not have to be the case. Many foods have anti-inflammatory properties. The book emphasizes minimizing pro-inflammatory foods while increasing anti-inflammatory foods.

3. Refocus the fuel: To lose weight consistently and permanently, your body must change its energy source to rely more

on fat as fuel rather than glucose (which is typically supplied by carb-heavy meals). If you do not burn all of the glucose in your system, it gets stored as body fat. This metabolic fact inspired me to develop a nutritional plan that is 70% healthy fats, 20% lean protein, and 10% quality carbohydrates. This ratio achieves three significant metabolic feats: It stimulates the body's fat-burning mechanisms. It helps the body break the addiction to sugar and processed carbohydrates. It also refocuses your diet on healthy fats, protein, and carbohydrates.

Chapter 1

Midlife changes

Our bodies are always evolving from the moment we are born until the day we die. This is a natural component of aging that no one can avoid. But, the changes that occur in women in their forties are unique and frequently unsettling. We're suddenly experiencing bizarre symptoms such as heat flashes and an accumulation of strange, new weight gain around our midsections. Our skin might become extremely dry or wrinkled. Joint discomfort, hair loss, headaches, bloating, and increasing anxiety or depression are all possibilities. Sleep becomes difficult to come by. Sexual encounters can be painful. We were triggered by insignificant events. This might be happening to you right now. Certainly, your body is changing, but this is a normal part of life that all of us women go through, primarily due to hormone swings. This period of physical transition is divided into three stages: perimenopause, menopause, and postmenopause. They affect us in different ways. Let's go over what happens at each level.

Perimenopause

Perimenopause (the prefix peri- is Greek for "around" or "near") refers to the period before menopause when fertility declines and menstrual cycles become irregular, lasting from the first menstrual period to the first year after the last menstrual period. Perimenopause differs widely from woman to woman. It lasts three to four years on average, but it can be as short as a few months before the last menstrual period or as long as a decade. Some women are bothered by hot flashes or mood swings, and exhausted by heavy periods or insomnia, while others have none of these symptoms. Menstrual cycles might end abruptly or continue irregularly for years.

Confronting one's waning fertility can be a huge difficulty for someone considering a pregnancy.

Even for those who do not wish to become pregnant, early signs of menopause, such as hot flashes and fluctuating periods, can be perplexing. To help you understand what's going on, let's look at the midlife hormonal changes that are causing your symptoms.

What's Going on With My Body?

Hormonal Changes Explained

Hormones are chemicals that are created and released into the bloodstream by several specialized endocrine glands as well as the hypothalamus, a region of the brain. The pineal and pituitary glands are located near the brain, the thyroid gland is located in the neck, the adrenal gland and pancreas are located in the midsection, and the ovary [in women] and testes are located further down. Some cells in the body, such as those in adipose tissue, can produce hormones.)

Hormones go to cells and tissues throughout the body, where they have a tremendous impact on our health, emotions, and behaviors. The leading hormone throughout the menopausal transition is estrogen, which is produced or, as we will discover, is not reliably generated by the ovaries.

Perimenopause Symptoms

It can be difficult to distinguish between symptoms caused directly by perimenopausal hormone changes and symptoms caused by natural aging or in response to common midlife stressors such as children leaving home, changes in primary relationships or occupations, or illness or death of parents. Hot flashes, night sweats, and vaginal dryness have all been conclusively linked to perimenopause in studies, and menopausal hormone therapy efficiently cures these "core" symptoms, according to the study. Although there may be a definitive link between fluctuating or low estrogen levels and other symptoms commonly associated with perimenopause, such as sleep disturbance, mood swings, memory and concentration issues, low sex drive, and urinary complaints, current research has not conclusively proven this. Furthermore, there is debate concerning the efficacy of hormone therapy in treating some of these "secondary" symptoms. The primary perimenopause symptoms, however, frequently have concomitant consequences. Frequent, intense hot flashes can make it difficult to sleep and can also make you feel exhausted, anxious, irritable, and confused. Dryness in the vaginal area can make sex difficult and ultimately reduce a woman's desire for sex.

As a result, hormone therapy may also help with some of the secondary symptoms to the extent that it reduces the primary symptoms of menopause.

Night sweats and hot flashes

In Western nations, hot flashes are the most often reported perimenopause symptom among women. Studies show that up to 80% of American women, though numbers vary, have hot flashes at some point throughout the menopausal transition. The severity of hot flashes tends to peak in the first two years following a woman's last menstrual period, then gradually decrease over the next four to five years. About 10% of women, nevertheless, will experience hot flashes indefinitely, maybe for the remainder of their lives. Hot flashes are more common in women whose ovaries have undergone surgical removal or have been harmed by illnesses or treatments that impair the ovaries' capacity to produce hormones.

Even while one-hour episodes are not unheard of, hot flashes normally last between one and five minutes and come on suddenly. Women have a sensation of a hot wave sweeping across their face, neck, and chest. A minor hot flash might be compared to a momentary warmth, however, a severe hot flash can make one feel as though they are on fire from the inside out and are burning up. Hot flashes that are more intense cause flushing (reddening) of the skin, and excessive sweating, and are frequently followed by chills and clamminess. It's not unusual to have heart palpitations, dizziness, disorientation, worry, tension, or a hazy sense of dread.

Some females get upset just before they flash. Others describe tingling or itching feelings in their hands or fingers, or the feeling of insects crawling within or on top of their skin. Formication is the medical term for this creepy skin sensation, which comes from the Latin word for "ant."(Heart palpitations or formication can occasionally accompany hot flashes.) Flashing during an awkward situation, such as a speech, interview, romantic tryst, or while driving, can be very upsetting.

Hot flashes occur at varying rates. The average number of flashes each day is 3 to 4, but some women only encounter 3 to 4 in a week, while others may have 10 or more, plus some at night. Night sweats are a name given to hot flashes that occur in the early morning hours for a good reason. You might jump awake to discover your bedding and clothes covered in sweat. It can be challenging to relax and go back to sleep when your heart is racing. Being sleep deprived can cause anxiety and mood swings.

Insomnia

A common perimenopause complaint is sleep disturbance. It's unclear exactly how much hot flashes and night sweats interfere with sleep. While other women claim to sleep through their hot flashes, some claim to perspire so heavily that they drench their sheets and wake up. Women who don't have hot flashes or night sweats may nonetheless struggle with insomnia. While some women may have trouble falling asleep when they first go into bed, the more typical trend is for women to sleep for a few hours, wake up too early, and then have trouble getting back asleep. It is unknown if sleep disturbances that happen when hot flashes are not present are largely brought on by menopause's hormonal changes.

But aging-related decreases in other hormones, such as melatonin, can also be bad for sleep. The internal clock that regulates your sleep-wake cycle, the circadian clock, appears to be regulated by the pineal gland's production of melatonin. When everything is in order, your pineal gland releases melatonin when the light in the evening grows dim, telling you it's time to go to bed. Additionally, it stops producing when the sun comes up, causing your melatonin levels to skyrocket at dawn and waking you up.

Whatever its cause, insomnia is a bothersome issue that can make its sufferers tired, anxious, angry, and grumpy. Chronic sleep deprivation has also been linked to weight gain, high blood pressure, coronary heart disease, lowered immune function, poor memory and problem-solving skills, and diminished immune function.

Mood Change

In early perimenopause, when hormonal fluctuations are most erratic, moodiness or mood swings—feeling calm and content one minute but anxious, irritable, depressed, or discouraged the next appear to be more prevalent than in the years after menopause when ovarian hormones stabilize at a low level.

However, these emotional alterations typically do not satisfy the requirements for a formal diagnosis of major depression, a far more severe and incapacitating condition. Women without a history of major depression are no more likely to experience major depression during these years than at other times in their lives, even if they may be more susceptible to recurrences during perimenopause.

The main causes of mood disturbances during the menopausal transition seem to be stressful life conditions rather than hormonal changes. Even though the majority of us have dealt with a variety of life's curveballs at younger ages, we may still feel unprepared to handle the numerous difficulties that can appear in midlife, such as chronic illness in oneself or a family member; a failing marriage, divorce, or widowhood; changing dynamics with adolescents or adult children; worries about aging parents and increased caregiver responsibilities; career stress; financial pressures; and setting up a family.

Problems with Memory and Concentration

Women frequently lament short-term memory loss and attention issues during perimenopause. Age, not changing hormone levels, may be the source of several of these problems. However, several perimenopause-related factors, such as tension about heavy bleeding, persistently intense hot flashes, sleep loss, or mood changes, as well as excessive worry about memory itself, can undoubtedly cause a lack of focus. You're not the first person to enter a space or dial a number only to forget what or who they were looking for. Remain calm. It occurs to many of us. Most of the time, mild memory deterioration associated with age does not portend the development of more severe cognitive issues, such as Alzheimer's disease.

Low sexual arousal

There are several reasons why sexual desire can diminish as we age. Reduced estrogen or circulatory changes brought on by aging could diminish blood flow to the genitals and lessen sensation. As previously mentioned, vaginal thinning or dryness can make sex uncomfortable. Additionally, women with sleep issues may feel too worn out to be interested in sex. Urinary incontinence can make people feel embarrassed, which makes sex less appealing. Reduced sex drive can also result from worries about physical attractiveness and body image.

It has long been believed that low blood testosterone levels in both men and women cause poor sexual desire because sex drive may be more strongly correlated with testosterone than with estrogen.

Incontinence of the urine

Urinary incontinence affects 30 to 40% of women between the ages of 50 and 64, compared to no more than 5% of men of the same age. Due to fundamental anatomical variations between the sexes and the consequences of vaginal childbirth on pelvic tissues, women are disproportionately affected.

The lining of the urethra, the tube that empties the bladder of pee, may thin as a result of decreased estrogen or it may contribute to this thinning. The muscles that surround the pelvis may become weaker as we age. The desire to urinate more frequently, unexpected urges to urinate even when your bladder is not full, the difficulty to hold your urine long enough to reach the bathroom, urine leaks when laughing, sneezing, or coughing, and pain when urinating are all signs of a problem. A urinary tract infection frequently causes painful urination.

Wrinkles and Skin Changes

In midlife, a lot of women start to get dry, wrinkled, or sagging skin. It is doubtful that a drop in estrogen is the main cause of these issues, despite some data to the contrary. Your genes play a big role in how quickly your skin ages and years of excessive sun exposure and cigarette smoke also speed up the process.

Headaches

Headaches have been associated with hormonal shifts. Younger women frequently complain of "menstrual migraines" around the time of their periods, and some migraine sufferers claim that their migraines grow better when pregnant. Instead of a persistently low level, experts think that fluctuations in the blood estrogen levels may be the cause of migraines. Some perimenopausal women may be more prone to migraines due to the unpredictable hormonal changes that occur before menopause.

Smoke and pollen, alcohol, lack of sleep, specific foods like chocolate and aged cheeses, stress, and other things can all cause headaches of various types. When hormone levels are in flux, these causes may cause headaches more frequently. For women who have experienced regular menstrual migraines, perimenopause may see an aggravation of the condition. However, some women claim that following menopause, their headaches grow better or even stop.

further signs or other additional symptoms appear during perimenopause, and you are rarely informed of them. For example

Breast pain

Dry eyes

High cholesterol levels

Having dry or itchy skin

high blood pressure

Palpitations

Panic attacks

Constipation

Dry mouth

Menopause

When you go 12 months without having a period, you have reached menopause. Although it can appear before or beyond this age, it is most common between the ages of 45 and 55. Weight gain might worsen throughout menopause and be more difficult to lose. Each ovary contains roughly a million eggs when a woman is born. About 300,000 eggs are still present during puberty, and no active eggs are remaining by menopause.

Your ovaries begin to change around the age of 35 to 40, and estrogen and progesterone are no longer produced in the same regular manner. The hormone release becomes irregular, fluctuating between being less and more frequent. Your ovaries' egg reserves begin to diminish more quickly at this time as well. Your body eventually stops ovulating (producing an egg from an ovary), which results in a decrease in estrogen. Your monthly periods will eventually stop, which will cause menopause.

You will also experience more acute hunger signals, which make you want to eat more food and inevitably raise your chances of gaining weight. Women gain between 12 and 15 pounds on average between the ages of 45 and 55. Although there are correlations between the age at menopause and specific demographic, physical, and genetic factors, it is impossible to determine when a specific woman will go through menopause.

Menopause can also be brought on by medical procedures (such as radiation therapy or chemotherapy) that result in the termination of ovarian function or surgical operations that require the removal of both ovaries.

Many women already stop menstruation before menopause, including those who have undergone certain surgical operations (such as a hysterectomy or the surgical removal of their uterine lining), use specific hormonal contraceptives, and use other medications that induce irregular or nonexistent periods. They could still go through additional menopausal-related changes. Your feelings regarding menopause may be influenced by your cultural heritage. Menopause is viewed as a social milestone in some cultures that carries with it experience and wisdom. It could be interpreted negatively in Western societies as a symptom of aging. Additionally, even among friends, talking about menopause and its changes may be frowned upon.

You might believe that menopause ushers in a rich, novel, and perhaps even liberated stage of life if you come from a society where older women are valued as community and family leaders. Menopause will be a time of liberation from the possibility of pregnancy for some women, but it may also be a sad period for those who desired children but were unable to have them.

Post menopause

When a woman hasn't had a period for more than a year following menopause, that period is known as postmenopause.

Health following menopause
Menopause symptoms may have subsided or gone totally in postmenopause, but some people continue to experience them for longer.

However, the change in your body's hormone levels is a reminder to continue taking care of your health and well-being and to pay attention to what your body is telling you.

Following menopause, there may be an increased chance of developing certain medical disorders, including urinary tract infections (UTIs), osteoporosis, and cardiovascular disease (heart disease). Therefore, it's crucial to lead a healthy lifestyle and take frequent cancer screenings like the cervical (smear test), and breast.

cardiovascular Disease

As a result of menopause, your risk of cardiovascular disease rises when your body's estrogen levels fall. Your risk of having coronary heart disease or stroke may increase as a result of the narrowing of the coronary arteries.

Osteoporosis

Due to the decreasing levels of estrogen in their bodies, women who have experienced menopause are more likely to develop osteoporosis, which is characterized by fragile bones that can break more easily.

By consistently exercising, you can lower your risk of developing osteoporosis by taking hormone replacement therapy, which prevents the weakening of your bones and becomes more effective the longer it is taken. a balanced diet rich in calcium-rich foods like low-fat milk and yogurt, as well as weight-bearing and resistance exercises, quitting smoking, cutting back on alcohol, and taking calcium and/or vitamin D supplements.

Changes in vaginal discharge and dryness

Postmenopause is often accompanied by changes in vaginal discharge or increased dryness in and around the genitalia. Vaginal atrophy, a disorder where the vaginal walls narrow, maybe the cause of these symptoms.

15% of people have vaginal atrophy before menopause and 40% to 57% do so later. The following are typical signs of vaginal atrophy:

vaginal dryness

burning or itching around the genitals

pain during vaginal intercourse

a yellow-tinged vaginal discharge

spotting or bleeding

Additionally, vaginal discharge may become less frequent after menopause, raising the possibility of unpleasant sex. Estrogen and progesterone, which are important for healthy discharge and natural lubrication, have fallen sharply, which causes a decrease in natural vaginal flow.

Your postmenopausal years will be significantly healthier and more fulfilling as a result of the nutrition and lifestyle techniques you will learn about in this book.

Consider the possibilities of all that time! If you have children, menopause typically occurs when they are starting or have started their own adult life. This gives you more time to spend on yourself and the chance to rethink your plans for the future. You have time to find your passions, follow them, establish a business, work for a cause, write, create art, spend more time with loved ones, take in nature, run for government, or pursue any other activity that matters to you.

Anything! In that sense, view menopause as a privilege. It implies that you have experienced a life that many others do not, for a variety of reasons. For instance, I make a big deal out of my birthday every year since I'm so appreciative to be alive despite having a few wrinkles, gray hair, and creaky joints.

Consider this time as an opportunity to get to know oneself better. Be deliberate in your decisions rather than feeling horrible about this stage of life and upset with the symptoms. Focus on the positives rather than the negatives after learning more about your body and what, in terms of food, exercise, or relationships, works and doesn't for you. This could be the best time of your life if you can change the way you view menopause and follow the advice in this book.

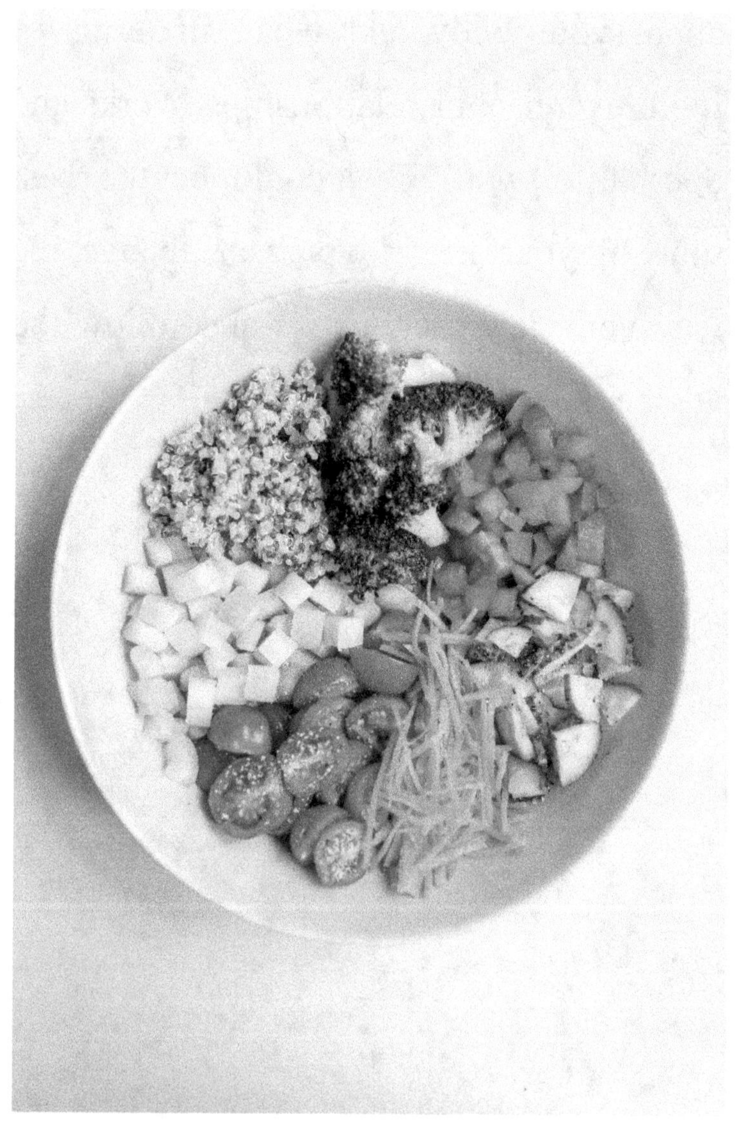

Chapter 2

Taking control of your hormones

Weight gain is a problem that goes beyond what you eat or how much exercise you get. Your hormones may also have an impact on it, and vice versa. It may be beneficial for you to raise these concerns with your doctor if you've observed hormonal changes or weight swings. Understanding how your body functions, particularly how many of its seemingly independent activities are interconnected, is one of the greatest ways to get there.

The link between your hormones and weight

A person's weight increase or loss is frequently directly attributed to changing their eating or activity routine. You can get upset with yourself and start working out more if you suspect you've put on a few pounds.

On the other hand, if the scale indicates that you are heavier than usual, you might applaud yourself for improving your diet. While many people don't even consider it, bigger weight fluctuations are sometimes caused by hormonal changes or imbalances.

Studies have shown that hormonal fluctuations can affect your appetite, including how much food you consume and what kinds of cravings you have. Depending on their balance, they may even make you store more or less fat in your body.

Because of this, telling someone to "exercise and eat right" isn't necessarily enough to make a genuine change in their life, especially if hormones play a role in how much weight they can gain or lose.

Your Hormones and You

Your body uses hormones as chemical messengers. Numerous glands and organs, such as the intestines, ovaries, adrenal glands, and brain, constantly release different hormones. They influence the behavior of cells all across the body. To maintain equilibrium, they communicate frequently with one another and other substances in the body.

Hormones are in charge when it comes to your weight and other perimenopause and menopause symptoms.

Along with other things, they regulate things like metabolism, appetite, hunger, and food cravings. Your attempts to lose weight may be thwarted if certain hormones are out of balance. Not only are chronic inflammation, stroke, Diabetes, heart disease, and obesity connected to low levels of specific hormones.

Fortunately, controlling your hormones can help you avoid gaining weight and combat inflammation. With the nutritionally based techniques, you'll learn in this book, you can do all of this.

These hormones, and especially regulating them with eating, are the solution to hormonal weight gain and other midlife symptoms.

Insulin

When it comes to weight gain and loss, insulin is one of the most crucial hormones. Insulin, which is produced by the pancreas, either stores blood sugar or uses it, depending on what your body requires at the time. A significant amount of insulin is released into the bloodstream following a hefty meal. Additionally, it enters the bloodstream when necessary during the day to maintain blood sugar levels.

Fat storage is one of these hormones' important roles. Insulin determines how much fat will be stored and how much will be used for energy. Insulin resistance is a disorder that is connected to an increase in blood sugar as well as persistently higher insulin levels and is brought on by long-term high levels of insulin.

It is essential to stop this insulin imbalance since it causes weight gain and, eventually, type 2 diabetes. Obesity and metabolic syndrome are frequently the sad results when insulin levels remain high for a long time.

What you can do: Cut back on consuming too many items that raise insulin levels.

How can we maintain balanced insulin levels? The first step is to quit overeating. Insulin resistance is a well-known result of overeating, especially when we consume quantities of food that are unhealthy for our bodies and minds. When we consume excessive amounts of sugar, fast food, and processed carbohydrates, insulin malfunctions. Weight gain and mild inflammation are caused by these high insulin levels. According to one study, eating too many of these items in a short period causes insulin resistance and weight gain.

Restricting carbohydrates in your diet may also be a good idea. A low-carb diet avoids metabolic syndrome and the associated insulin resistance. Other research indicates that taking omega-3 fatty acids from fatty fish, drinking green tea, and getting enough protein all help maintain healthy insulin levels.

A diet that helps keep insulin levels normal

minimal carbohydrates. You can eat carbs, but limit your intake and make informed choices. Avoid processed foods like white bread and pasta in favor of the carbohydrates found in fruits, vegetables, whole grains, legumes, and low-fat dairy. Even preferable are whole grains that haven't been processed into flour. So instead of toast for the morning, opt for oats.

healthy protein. Getting enough protein is important, but not at the expense of fat. Beef, lamb, and pork should be kept to a minimum.

without the skin: chicken or turkey

fish include salmon, sardines, and albacore tuna

Cheese with less fat and egg whites

Plant proteins such as those found in beans, lentils, and nut butter.

wholesome fats. Lowering insulin resistance can be achieved by substituting healthy fats for saturated and trans fats. That entails consuming more olive, sunflower, and sesame oils while consuming less meat, full-fat dairy, and butter.

dairy products with low fat. You can get calcium, protein, and fewer calories by consuming low-fat milk and plain, nonfat yogurt. Additionally, numerous studies demonstrate that low-fat dairy reduces insulin resistance.

If you're used to eating full-fat, dial it back gradually. So before moving to skim milk, you might want to try 1% or 2% milk first. high in fiber. More than 50 grams of fiber per day contribute to blood sugar regulation. Oatmeal, broccoli, black beans, lentils, and black beans are all high in fiber.

Foods to Avoid

processed foods, which can contain extra salt, sugar, and fat. It has probably been processed if it arrives in cans, cartons, wrappers, or other packaging.

Trans fats and saturated fats may increase insulin resistance. These are mostly found in foods cooked in partially hydrogenated oils as well as animal products like meats and cheese.

Drinks with added sugar, such as soda, fruit juice, iced tea, and vitamin water, might cause weight gain.

Leptin

Another hormone that is crucial to comprehend if we're concerned about preserving a healthy weight is leptin. Leptin is often referred to as the hormone that suppresses appetite. Leptin, which is produced in fat cells, is responsible for making you feel full. Your brain listens to it when you're hungry or full. When your leptin levels are in check, you won't overeat because you'll feel satisfied for hours after eating a well-balanced meal. Like insulin, leptin detests improper foods. Have you ever noticed how soon you feel hungry and depleted after eating processed meals and sweets? Leptin resistance develops over time as a result of eating processed foods and trans fats.

What you must understand regarding leptin resistance

Leptin levels rise as your body develops a resistance to it. When leptin levels are checked in overweight people, they frequently turn out to be up to four times higher than usual. Once leptin levels have built up resistance, it is quite challenging to restore balance.

Due to decreased brain-leptin communication caused by leptin resistance, your brain may not recognize when you are full and may instead instruct your body to continue eating. It's as though your brain misinterprets your leptin resistance for starvation.

Let's discuss diet, drink, and supplements to treat leptin resistance or stop it from occurring to you in the first place. Your diet has an impact on everything in your body, including leptin. You should eat less sugar because it can dramatically increase your body's leptin levels. Leptin resistance can also be avoided or reduced in the following ways:

eating an anti-inflammatory diet

Adding anti-inflammatory fish oil to your diet

establishing a regular exercise schedule

Regularly getting the restorative sleep

Estrogen

Estrogen, which is made in the ovaries, is essential for the healthiest operation of all female reproductive organs. Estrogen encourages fat storage so that women can have healthy pregnancies. The proper quantity of fat aids in the execution of female reproductive activities when estrogen levels are balanced. However, weight gain frequently happens when there is either insufficient or excessive estrogen.

Women who are overweight and those who are in the first trimester of pregnancy often have high estrogen levels. Then there is menopause, which is marked by a significant drop in estrogen, and perimenopause. Some women choose hormone replacement therapy during this time to supplement their declining estrogen levels.

Foods that help manage Estrogen

1. Cruciferous veggies

Because they contain indole-3-carbinol, a substance with estrogen-reducing properties, cruciferous vegetables are among the most significant nutrients that suppress estrogen.

In other words, cruciferous vegetables like cauliflower, broccoli, bok choy, and Brussels sprouts can lessen the amount of estrogen that males produce.

It's also important to note that eating these vegetables can reduce your risk of developing prostate cancer.

2. Curcumin and turmeric

Turmeric is a spice that contains curcumin, which gives it a recognizable, vivid yellow hue. There is evidence that curcumin may lower estrogen levels.

Additionally, a high curcumin intake can raise testosterone levels. Men who want to naturally enhance their testosterone levels should pay special attention to this.

While additional research is required, the available data on these foods that block estrogen are encouraging. The best part about turmeric is that incorporating it into your diet to reduce estrogen is simple. Additionally, there are nutritional supplements that contain turmeric and curcumin.

3. Fish with fat

Fatty fish like salmon and mackerel, which are high in Omega-3 fatty acids, zinc, and vitamin D, are also foods that lower estrogen levels.

4. A plant-based diet

Those who follow plant-centric eating patterns typically have estrogen levels that are lower than those who don't. They are also less likely to experience health issues brought on by an excess of estrogen.

It's crucial to keep in mind that eating a plant-based diet doesn't require you to become a vegan unless you want to. Make sure that plant foods make up more than half of the food on your plate.

Cortisol

Cortisol, also referred to as the stress hormone, is produced by the adrenal glands. It is created far too frequently in the modern era despite being necessary for survival. Cortisol is produced in the bloodstream whenever your body or mind considers itself to be under stress. The issue is that we experience stress far too frequently these days, which causes our bodies to produce more cortisol than is healthy.

How is this cortisol overproduction connected to weight gain? The first is that eating too much is associated with elevated cortisol. Have you ever noticed how you eat under pressure? Cortisol levels that were higher than usual were connected to overeating and weight gain, according to a study. Another study relates an increase in abdominal fat to elevated cortisol levels.

foods that assist in maintaining a healthy level of cortisol

bitter chocolate: The high flavonoid content of dark chocolate has been demonstrated to reduce the release of cortisol by the adrenal glands' responsiveness to stress.

whole grains. Whole grains, as opposed to refined grains, are high in fiber and plant-based polyphenols which might benefit gut health and stress levels.

lentils and legumes: They include a lot of fiber, which promotes intestinal health and regulates blood sugar.

fruit and veggie wholes: Antioxidants and polyphenolic chemicals are abundant in whole fruits and vegetables, helping to fend off free radicals that damage cells.

Herbal tea: L-theanine, a soothing substance found in green tea, has been associated with lowered stress levels and improved mental clarity.

Prebiotics as well as probiotics: Friendlier, symbiotic bacteria can be found in foods like yogurt, sauerkraut, and kimchi. These bacteria are fed by prebiotics such as soluble fiber. Better gut and mental health are associated with both probiotics and prebiotics.

healthy fats. Better physical and mental health are linked to diets high in unsaturated fat and low in saturated fat. Omega-3 fatty acids in particular have the strongest associations with stress reduction and brain function. Nuts, seeds, and fatty fish are excellent sources.

Water: It is now even more crucial to stay hydrated throughout the day because dehydration has been associated with a transient rise in cortisol levels.

Ghrelin

Leptin and ghrelin are fundamentally antagonistic hormones. The hunger hormone sends a signal to your hypothalamus, alerting it that your stomach is empty and that you need to eat. Its principal function is to increase appetite. Ghrelin levels are often highest before meals and lowest afterward. Curiously, studies show that obese individuals have lower ghrelin levels yet are more susceptible to its effects. This sensitivity could make someone overeat.

Advice on controlling ghrelin levels

The fact that calorie restriction frequently raises ghrelin levels and makes you hungry is one reason why losing weight might be challenging. Additionally, leptin levels drop and metabolism tends to slow down.

As a result, the following advice for reducing ghrelin to aid in appetite suppression:

preserve healthy body weight. Your sensitivity to ghrelin may grow as a result of obesity, which would therefore increase your hunger.

Make an effort to get quality rest. Increases in ghrelin, overeating, and weight gain can result from lack of sleep.

Eat consistently: Ghrelin levels are at their peak just before a meal, so pay attention to your hunger cues and eat when it comes.

foods that assist maintain a healthy level of ghrelin

Foods high in protein: Protein can make you feel satisfied and full, which can help control your ghrelin levels. Lean meat, fish, eggs, dairy products, and legumes are all excellent sources of protein.

Foods high in fiber: Fiber can help you feel full for extended periods by slowing down digestion. Fruits, vegetables, whole grains, nuts, and seeds are among the foods high in fiber.

Fats that are good for you: Fats that are good for you, including those in nuts, seeds, avocados, and fatty fish, can help you feel full and control your appetite.

Water: Drinking enough water can help control ghrelin levels by keeping you hydrated. In actuality, humans occasionally confuse thirst with hunger, so drinking water might help limit mindless snacking.

Low-glycemic index foods: Foods with a low glycemic index, like whole grains, legumes, and non-starchy vegetables, can help regulate blood sugar levels and lessen appetite.

Chapter 3

Intermittent Fasting

Fasting is becoming increasingly trendy. Going for hours at a time without meals is undoubtedly more normal nowadays, and is even considered trendy by some. However, like with any health trend, it is critical to understand how your choices are influencing your body and, above all, to ensure you are not causing harm. The benefits of calorie restriction on health and life span are widely recognized. Fasting has been utilized for thousands of years for spiritual and health benefits, and it has recently gained popularity due to celebrity endorsements of intermittent fasting, sometimes known as the '5:2 fast diet' or the 16:8!

Although nutritional advice has traditionally emphasized eating regular low-fat meals, the 5:2's counterintuitive approach to weight management has drawn thousands of women. Fasting for weight loss is a well-kept secret in the nutrition world, but it is not always clear how to do so safely and successfully. Intermittent fasting is a way of eating that is simple and easy to practice. It involves adjusting your meal times to fit your lifestyle and weight loss goals. It is nothing more than a system that alternates between periods of not eating and periods of eating. Sounds weird, but don't we do this all the time

You have participated in a fast if you have ever eaten a meal in the evening, then gone to bed, woken up in the morning, and eaten breakfast. The time when you sleep at night is essentially a fast. However, eating breakfast and two additional meals with snacks in between has become the standard approach to meal management, the system that we are all told is the greatest and healthiest way to eat. For intermittent fasting to be effective, we must consider stretching out those 'fasting' intervals, which may be daily, or possibly a longer fast a couple of days a week, depending on the 'IF protocol' you adopt. What's great about intermittent fasting is that, in addition to giving a sustained, effective strategy to lose fat and enhance your body, it appears to work incredibly well for those who have struggled for years, if not decades, to lose weight and improve their health. This entails a 16-hour fast (evening, overnight, and morning) followed by an 8-hour eating window, usually from lunchtime until early evening. To conclude, Intermittent Fasting is an eating regimen in which you alternate between times of not eating and periods of eating methodically, with the non-eating intervals usually being somewhat longer than you would normally 'fast' while eating a standard three meals a day.

The advantages of intermittent fasting are numerous and include both physiological and psychological gains.

The Advantages of Intermittent Fasting for Women in Their Mid-Life

Intermittent fasting has several advantages, including physiological and psychological benefits.

As women approach their forties, they usually experience several physical and psychological changes. Intermittent fasting is one method that is becoming increasingly popular among women at this stage of their lives. This dietary pattern, which alternates between fasting and eating times, has shown promise in terms of overall health and well-being. In this section, we'll look at intermittent fasting as it relates to women in their forties and fifties, as well as its potential benefits, limitations, and useful implementation tips.

Hormonal balance: Intermittent fasting may help balance hormones like insulin, cortisol, and growth hormone, which may help regulate hormones like weight gain, mood swings, and hot flashes. Hormonal variations are prevalent during midlife.

Weight management: Many women may be concerned about weight increases in their middle years. By promoting fat burning, lowering insulin resistance, and helping to regulate calorie intake, intermittent fasting can help with weight management.

Improved Metabolism: As we age, our metabolisms can slow down, making weight loss more difficult. By boosting metabolic rate and accelerating fat oxidation, intermittent fasting may help healthy weight management.

Cellular Repair and Anti-aging Benefits:

Fasting triggers and intermittent fasting may help balance hormones such as insulin, cortisol, and growth hormone, which may help manage hormones such as weight gain, mood swings, and hot flashes. Hormonal fluctuations are common in midlife.

Mental Clarity and Brain Health: Some research suggests that intermittent fasting may boost cognitive performance and brain function, benefiting memory, focus, and overall mental clarity.

Understanding Middle-Aged Women's Nutritional Needs

Women's bodies alter physiologically and hormonally as they reach middle age. These modifications may have a substantial impact on their nutritional requirements and general health. Middle-aged women must prioritize a balanced diet that meets their individual needs. Women can promote their well-being, manage their weight, lower their risk of chronic diseases, and improve their quality of life by understanding and meeting these dietary needs. The purpose of this essay is to shed light on the necessary nutrients and dietary considerations for middle-aged women.

Calcium and Vitamin D: As women get older, their estrogen levels drop, putting them at an increased risk of developing osteoporosis. Adequate calcium and vitamin D intake are critical for bone health maintenance. Calcium can be obtained from dairy products, leafy green vegetables, fortified plant-based milk replacements, and calcium supplements. Vitamin D can also be gotten from fatty fish, fortified dairy or plant-based milk, and sun exposure.

Iron: Iron deficiency is becoming more common in middle-aged women as a result of variables such as monthly blood loss and impaired iron absorption. Iron is required for oxygen transport as well as the prevention of weariness and weakness. Lean meats, chicken, fish, legumes, fortified cereals, and dark leafy greens are all good sources of iron. Iron-rich diets with vitamin C sources, such as citrus fruits or peppers, are recommended to improve iron absorption.

Fiber: Because metabolism slows with age, middle-aged women are more prone to weight gain and digestive difficulties. Including a suitable amount of dietary fiber in their diet can help control bowel motions, maintain a healthy weight, and minimize the risk of heart disease and type 2 diabetes. Fiber is abundant in whole grains, fruits, vegetables, legumes, and nuts.

Omega-3 Fatty Acids: Omega-3 fatty acids are essential for heart health, decreasing inflammation, and supporting brain function. As women become older, their risk of heart disease rises, making omega-3s even more crucial. Omega-3 fatty acids are abundant in fatty fish such as salmon and sardines, flaxseeds, chia seeds, walnuts, and algae-based supplements.

Phytoestrogens: these are plant chemicals that can mimic estrogen in the body. They may help decrease menopausal symptoms and lower the risk of some diseases related to hormonal changes. Soy products such as tofu and tempeh, flaxseeds, sesame seeds, and legumes are high in phytoestrogens.

Antioxidants and phytochemicals: Middle-aged women should consume more antioxidant-rich foods to battle oxidative stress and lower their risk of chronic diseases. Colorful fruits and vegetables, such as berries, oranges, carrots, spinach, and kale, are high in vitamins, minerals, and phytochemicals, all of which support good health.

Water: Hydration is important at any age, but it becomes even more important as women age. Dehydration can cause weariness, cognitive deterioration, and bodily function impairment. Middle-aged women should drink plenty of water throughout the day and restrict their intake of sugary beverages.

Intermittent Fasting Approaches

TRF (Time-Restricted Feeding): TRF entails limiting your daily eating window to a set period, often between 8 and 10 hours, and fasting for the other 14 to 16 hours of the day. For example, you could eat all of your meals between 12 p.m. and 8 p.m., and then fast until noon the next day. This strategy is simple to adopt and adaptable to individual schedules. TRF is frequently regarded as a beginner-friendly technique for intermittent fasting.

Alternate-Day Fasting (ADF): This is the practice of alternating between fasting days and regular eating days. On days when you are fasting, your calorie intake is often limited to 500–600 calories, but on days when you are eating normally, there are no restrictions on what you can eat. The alternating nature of the fasting regimen makes this method more difficult for certain people. It might be appropriate for people who prefer longer fasts and have regular eating schedules.

5:2 Diet: The 5:2 diet calls for eating regularly five days a week while limiting calories to 500–600 calories on two separate days. It is typical to divide the calories between two short meals on fasting days. This strategy offers more flexibility than alternate-day fasting because it generally permits regular eating. To prevent a string of consecutive fasting days and to guarantee a balanced nutritional intake, it is crucial to choose fasting days carefully.

Extended Fasting: Extended fasting entails going without food for longer periods, usually longer than 24 hours. This might vary in length from a single day to many days, depending on the aims and skills of each person. Before attempting a lengthy fast, it is advised to obtain advice from a healthcare provider or certified nutritionist because it involves careful planning and monitoring. For beginners or people who have certain medical conditions, it is typically not advised.

It's crucial to remember that while intermittent fasting may be a useful technique for managing weight and may have health advantages, it may not be appropriate for everyone. Before beginning an intermittent fasting routine, people with underlying health concerns, women who are pregnant or nursing, and those who have a history of disordered eating should use caution and speak with a healthcare provider. As with any dietary strategy, it's critical to concentrate on eating a well-balanced diet during mealtimes, staying hydrated, and tuning into your body signals of hunger and fullness.

Approach to Fasting for Women It's important to carefully evaluate your personal health, lifestyle, and goals when deciding how to fast for middle-aged women. Weight loss, enhanced insulin sensitivity, and increased cellular repair are just a few advantages of fasting. Before making any significant dietary or fasting-related adjustments, it's crucial to exercise caution when fasting and speak with a healthcare provider. When choosing the best fasting strategy, keep the following elements in mind:

Health Status: It's important to evaluate your present state of health before beginning any fasting regimen. Women in their middle years may experience particular health issues like hormonal shifts, metabolic problems, or pre-existing diseases like diabetes or cardiovascular disease. To ensure a safe fasting method, consulting with a healthcare expert will assist identify any potential hazards or modifications required.

Lifestyle and Schedule: When deciding on a fasting strategy, take into account your daily schedule, professional commitments, and personal obligations. There are several approaches, including alternate-day fasting, time-restricted meals, and periodic protracted fasting. Choose a strategy that fits your lifestyle to make it simpler to continuously follow the fasting protocol.

Objectives and Goals: Establish your fasting objectives. Are you primarily interested in weight loss, higher energy levels, or other health benefits? Understanding your objectives can assist lead you in picking the most suited fasting approach. For instance, if losing weight is your main objective, you may want to try intermittent fasting or a lengthier fasting time. Periodic protracted fasting or time-restricted food may be an option if general health and longevity are your top priorities.

Gradual Implementation: It's normally advised to begin slowly and lengthen your fasts over time if you're new to fasting. This strategy lowers the possibility of negative effects while allowing your body to adjust to the changes. You can start with a shorter fasting window, like 12–14 hours, and then progressively increase it based on your needs.

Nutritional Needs: It's crucial to make sure you are getting the nutrients you need, particularly while starting a fasting routine. Middle-aged women have particular nutritional needs, including iron, calcium, and vitamin D, which are crucial for bone health and addressing any potential deficiency issues. During your eating windows, choose nutrient-dense meals, and think about speaking with a certified dietitian to make sure you're getting enough nourishment while fasting.

Monitoring and Modification: Pay attention to your body's cues and keep track of how you feel while fasting. If you encounter any negative side effects, such as weakness, severe hunger, or dizziness, it could be necessary to change your fasting strategy. Be willing to alter your fasting schedule or seek advice from a nutritionist or healthcare provider to determine the best course of action for your particular requirements.

Intermittent fasting dangers and implications for middle-aged women

Factors to bear in mind before embarking on intermittent fasting

While Intermittent Fasting has grown in popularity due to its potential health benefits, such as weight loss and improved metabolic health, there are some hazards and factors to bear in mind, particularly for middle-aged women. Here are a few examples:

Hormonal variations: Women in their forties and fifties may already be experiencing hormonal fluctuations as a result of perimenopause or menopause. Intermittent fasting can also affect hormone levels, potentially resulting in irregular periods, mood swings, or increased stress. Any changes must be monitored and discussed with a healthcare provider

Nutritional deficiencies: If the eating period is too short or the fasting phase is too protracted, IF can reduce the window for obtaining key nutrients. Middle-aged women have specific nutrient needs, such as calcium and vitamin D for bone health. It is critical to maintain a balanced diet during eating intervals to avoid deficits.

Blood sugar control: Middle-aged women may be more likely to develop insulin resistance or type 2 diabetes. While intermittent fasting can aid in blood sugar regulation, it can also cause hypoglycemia (low blood sugar) in some people. Monitoring blood sugar levels and changing fasting procedures as needed are recommended.

Bone health: Osteoporosis is more common in postmenopausal women. Long-term fasting or insufficient food intake during eating times can further raise this risk. While intermittent fasting, it's crucial to get enough calcium, vitamin D, and other nutrients that maintain bone health.

Disordered eating pattern Intermittent fasting may set off disordered eating habits or make pre-existing eating disorders, like binge eating or restrictive eating, worse. Women in their middle years who have a history of disordered eating should approach IF cautiously and seek expert advice.

Medication interactions: For best absorption and effectiveness, several medications call for timing the consumption of meals. To make sure that their medication schedule fits with their fasting and eating periods, women taking drugs should speak with their healthcare physician.

Psychological effects: Fasting may affect your mood and your ability to think clearly. Some women may get more irritable, have trouble focusing, or feel fatigued. Self-care, stress reduction, and upholding a balanced diet during mealtimes can all assist to lessen these impacts.

It's significant to remember that different people may react differently to intermittent fasting. Before beginning any fasting program, it is advised to speak with a healthcare provider or qualified nutritionist, especially for middle-aged women with unique health issues or medical disorders. They can offer customized guidance based on particular needs and assist in reducing potential dangers.

To successfully adopt intermittent fasting (IF), it is essential to set reasonable expectations and goals. Here are some important things to think about:

Choosing the Best Plan for You

After you've become acquainted with all of the recommended fasting ways for women, it's time to choose the one that speaks to you. It is critical to ensure that whichever fasting strategy you choose fits into your schedule. It is quite improbable that you will be able to sustain it long-term if it does not work with your current job and home routine. And here's the good news: you don't have to stick to any of the plans exactly. Combine elements from many schedules to build a timetable that works for you. Intermittent fasting allows for a lot of flexibility, and as long as you're feeling good while doing it, you don't have to worry about doing it exactly. Rigid regulations might exacerbate stress rather than alleviate it. You must enjoy what you are doing to some extent or you will never be able to remain with it.

Creating Your Fasting Schedule

Once you've decided on the style of intermittent fasting you wish to practice, the next step is to plan out your fasting schedule and write it down. Please do not skip this section. According to research, laying down a schedule increases the likelihood that you will keep to it. And if you can view your schedule every day, you'll gain extra points. Hang a kitchen wall calendar or put your weekly or monthly schedules on a large dry-erase board that you can update in real-time. If you're performing time-restricted fasting, you'll need to determine when you'll stop eating, how long your fasting window will last, and when you'll resume eating. For example, if you decide to stop eating at 7 p.m. and your fasting window is fourteen hours long, your schedule will look something like this:

Feeding window: 9a.m. to 7p.m. (you will eat all of your meals during this period) Fasting window: 7p.m. to 9a.m. (you'll stop eating dinner at 7p.m. every night and won't eat again until 9a.m the next morning) Because time-restricted fasting is often done every day of the week, after you figure out these figures, you'll simply stick to the same diet as long as you're feeling well and seeing results. If you follow a different fasting schedule, such as alternate-day fasting or 5:2, all you need to do is determine which days will be your eating days and which days will be your fasting days. For example, you might fast on Tuesdays, Thursdays, and Saturdays and eat normally on other days if you practice alternate-day fasting.

Maintaining Your Fasting Schedule

Once you've found a fasting plan that works for you, try to stick to it every week, especially on weekends when your schedule may be a little more casual. Maintaining a consistent schedule not only allows your body to adjust and become accustomed to fasting, but it also helps balance your hormones and increases the likelihood of a favorable experience.

Of course, there will be occasions when something unexpected occurs, such as a party or an early brunch with friends. If these things happen and you want to indulge, by all means, do so, even if they happen on your fasting days. A few off-schedule days here and there won't derail your progress, and having fun and getting out is a crucial component of not being overly stressed. The overarching lesson here is to make sure you're following the same fasting schedule most of the time, but don't be too hard on yourself if you don't.

Making a Plan That Will Produce Results

The most important thing to remember when starting an Intermittent Fasting habit is that the best results come from having a long-term strategy. Fasting is not intended to be used for rapid or short-term weight loss. This is a one-way eating disorder. There is a distinction to be made between fasting and starvation. There is a distinction to be made between purposely avoiding eating in search of a miracle cure and Intermittent Fasting as a lifestyle choice. It is also important to note that it is essential to consult with a medical practitioner before making any big changes to your health.

Gather as much information as possible

Creating a plan is the ideal way for first-time fasters and anyone interested in trying Intermittent Fasting to get a good idea of how their body will react to longer fasting windows without worrying about negative side effects like excess fatigue that can occur with an abrupt switch to the program. This is especially true for individuals who have elected not to ease into fasting by cutting back on one meal or a couple of hundred calories at a time in the weeks preceding their first real fasting window. Before planning your first major fasting window or beginning an Intermittent Fasting plan, learn everything you can about fasting, fitness, diets that work with fasting schedules to maximize health benefits, and any other questions that may be causing concern, hesitation, or simply remain unanswered. The more information you have at your disposal, the easier it will be to develop a strategy that you can keep to while also providing the most health advantages with the fewest adverse effects.

Establish Your Motivation and Set Realistic Goals

Before beginning any diet or exercise plan, it is critical to understand why you want to make the change and everything that comes with it. Simply because a new health trend is sweeping the globe does not imply that it is the best option for everyone or that it will work for everyone. Any diet or exercise regimen demands adaptability, attention, determination, and sacrifice. This is one of the reasons why it is a good idea to consider, if not write down, your reasons for wanting to begin an Intermittent Fasting routine. This will not only help with goal setting, but it will also give an excellent source of support and inspiration on days when temptation calls or there has been a hiccup in your plans that has disrupted your fasting schedule. Once you've determined why you want to attempt Intermittent Fasting, it's time to define your health goals and expectations for the schedule you intend to begin. In one month, three months, six months, and a year, where do you want to be? Even if you are unsure how soon your body will adjust to Intermittent Fasting and any other programs you may be experimenting with (such as a specific diet or workout regimen), Setting goals before you begin your Intermittent Fasting plan gives you a starting point for goals and progress when it comes time to make schedule adjustments. Making a list of questions and then going to the internet, their local gym, or any healthcare professional to get the information they need to start moving forward is one step new runners may take to ease their planning and preparation stages.

Asking the Right Questions Before Beginning A Fasting Program

consider the following questions:

What are my short-term (three to six months) and long-term health goals (one year and beyond)?

This could be a specific number of pounds or inches lost as a result of Intermittent Fasting. It could also be something less particular in terms of fitness, such as getting fit enough to tackle a local trail or walking a marathon.

Have I chosen the best Intermittent Fasting approach for my unique needs and goals?

Is fasting the best option for me?
Have I spoken with my physician or another medical professional to ensure a safe transition into and long-term consistency withIntermittent Fasting?

Is the strategy I've devised feasible in terms of my present health status and existing conditions, as well as meeting my health objectives?

Have I assessed the advantages and disadvantages of beginning an Intermittent Fasting plan and determined what I can do to make the transition as simple as possible before beginning?

When these questions are thoroughly answered, each individual will have all they need to begin their initial steps towards success with an Intermittent Fasting lifestyle.

The gradual path is sometimes the best path to take.

Intermittent fasting entails adopting a new way of life that enhances overall health and wellness. As a result, easing into a personalized Intermittent Fasting regime has several advantages, including:

A less difficult or troublesome transition into a specific Intermittent Fasting plan. More time to observe how the body reacts to fasting as a normal part of life, allowing adjustments to be made to alleviate discomfort or eliminate potential harmful consequences. They have an easier time tweaking, fine-tuning, and changing their unique plan to combat adverse effects or maximize health advantages. Those who view fasting as a short treatment for a specific problem or disease will often see less progress and advantages than those who accept it as a lifestyle choice for the betterment of their overall health and fitness. It is natural to be excited at the beginning of any new health journey, but with Intermittent Fasting, the more time spent understanding the feelings and changes the body is communicating, the more likely a person is to see long-term success with their personalized (and constantly evolving) fasting plan.

Seek Professional Advice to Ensure Your Health and Safety

When it comes to diets, exercise, and fasting, the best advice to follow comes from a healthcare professional, preferably a personal physician who is already familiar with the participant's particular medical history and current health state. If a personal physician is not involved, a dietician or nutritionist can provide medical information regarding potential hazards as well as advice on how to maximize the benefits of Intermittent Fasting. That concludes the principles and essentials of Intermittent Fasting for ladies! All that remains is for you to create your personalized plan and begin your journey toward a healthy lifestyle supported by Intermittent Fasting.

Drink more water than you did before you began fasting.

One of the most common side effects experienced by men and women during the first week of a new or modified Intermittent Fasting strategy is dehydration. Any harmful effects of dehydration can be readily mitigated or avoided by simply drinking six to eight glasses of water every day.

Pay attention to hunger pangs, just like you did in the first week. They are frequently caused by thirst and dehydration rather than a lack of food. Another concern that many women notably express during the first week of a new fasting routine is difficulty sleeping (during the first three and five days on the new fast schedule). The good news is that following that, the majority of people (both men and women) who practice Intermittent Fasting as part of their regular lives reported deeper periods of sleep and faster times falling asleep each night as they adhered to their personalized fasting schedule.

In their first week of Intermittent Fasting, all new fasting participants should anticipate experiencing the following symptoms: Muscle ache or weakness Nausea, constipation, and other digestive issues Increased thirst and hunger A tendency to get easily distracted or to struggle to acquire or maintain attention

The best way to combat these issues and ensure that they do not impede personal health progress is to ensure that enough water is consumed even during fasting windows, enough calories are consumed during feeding windows, and the body is not put under undue strain until it has had time to adapt to a fluctuating eating and fasting schedule.

Pay Attention to Your Mind and Body

Over the Week Spend the additional non-fasting day of your first week mentally preparing for your next fast (the first fasting window of the next week) and another week of Intermittent Fasting for your health. This could be going for a contemplative walk or starting to meditate. For some, this just means unwinding and celebrating their first week of Intermittent Fasting. Some key questions to consider at the end of the first planned fasting week: How do I feel? What about physically, psychologically, and emotionally? Is there anything about my personalized fasting plan that I'm convinced isn't working right now? Is there anything I can see that has to be changed right away for my health? Is there anything that is making me unwell or endangering my general health?

Are there any symptoms I should keep an eye on in the second week to see whether they go away or if they indicate that something about the Intermittent Fasting strategy needs to be changed?

The best way to determine whether or not Intermittent Fasting will work for you and your long-term health goals is to listen to your mind and body, what they are trying to communicate, and how they react when diet, eating habits, or other health-related factors are changed.

Making an intermittent fasting plan Here's an example food schedule for 16:8 intermittent fasting:

Break your fast at 8:00 A.M

Begin your morning with a glass of water or herbal tea. Consume a nutrient-dense breakfast rich in healthy fats, protein, and fiber. Scrambled eggs with vegetables and avocado are two examples. Greek yogurt topped with berries and almonds. Oatmeal with chia seeds and almond butter on top.

Lunch at 12:00 P.M

Consume a well-balanced lunch that delivers important nutrients and keeps you going until your next meal. Grilled chicken breast or fish with roasted veggies is an example. Salad of quinoa or brown rice, mixed greens, grilled tofu, and a light vinaigrette.

Lentil soup with whole-grain bread and a green salad on the side.

Snack time at 3:00 P.M

Consume a healthy snack to maintain your energy levels. A handful of nuts (almonds, walnuts, or cashews) is a good choice. A piece of fruit (either an apple, a banana, or an orange). Greek yogurt or cottage cheese with honey drizzle and chopped almonds.

Dinner at 6:00 P.M

Dinner should be filling and well-rounded, with a concentration on lean protein, veggies, and whole grains. Grilled fish with steamed broccoli and quinoa is one example. Tofu or lean meat stir-fried with mixed vegetables and brown rice. Baked chicken breast served with roasted sweet potatoes and a salad on the side.

Evening snack (optional) at 7:30 P.M

If you need a tiny snack, go for something light and low in calories. Among the options are: Hummus on carrot sticks. A few cherry tomatoes topped with mozzarella cheese. A tiny serving of mixed berries.

8:00 PM: Begin fasting Finish your final meal of the day and begin your fast till the next morning. Remember to pay attention to your body's hunger and fullness cues and alter your schedule accordingly. Maintain hydration throughout the day and get medical advice before beginning any new diet or fasting plan.

BREAKFAST MEAL PLANS

Breakfast

1. Healthy Rainbow Acai Bowl

Preparation Time: 5 minutes

Cooking Time: 0 minutes

Servings: 2

Ingredients:

1/4 cup frozen raspberries

1/4 cup frozen blueberries

1/2 cup nonfat Greek yogurt

1 teaspoon chia seeds

1 teaspoon acai powder

1 teaspoon vanilla protein powder

1 mango, sliced

1 small orange, segmented

1 tablespoon pistachios, chopped, toasted

Directions: In a blender, blend berries, yogurt, chia seed, acai powder, and mango until very smooth; spoon into two serving bowls and top each with fresh blueberries, strawberries, bananas, oranges, and pistachios. Enjoy!

Nutrition:

Calories: 198

Total Fat: 2.9 g

Carbs: 11.5 g

Dietary Fiber: 6.4 g

Protein: 18.6 g

2. Eggs in a Hole

Preparation Time: 10 minutes

Cooking Time: 10 minutes

Servings: 2

Ingredients:

2 and ½ slices whole wheat bread

Olive oil Spray

Fresh ground Pepper

Hot sauce to taste

Salt to taste

2 and ½ ounces of avocado flesh, mashed

2 large eggs

Directions:

Take your bread slices and make a hole in the middle using a cookie cutter. Season avocado mash with salt and pepper. Take a skillet and place it over medium-low heat, grease with cooking spray. Place bread slices and a cut portion in the skillet. Break the egg into the hole of the bread, cook until the egg properly settles down, and season with more salt and pepper. Flip and cook the other side. Once done, transfer to a plate. Top the egg with avocado mash, hot sauce, and crumble bread (made from the cut piece). Enjoy!

Nutrition:

Calories: 229g

Fat: 23g

Carbohydrates: 10g

Protein: 12g

3. Baked Cinnamon-Orange French Toast

Preparation Time: 10 minutes

Cooking Time: 12 minutes

Servings: 4

Ingredients:

Nonstick cooking spray

3 large eggs

½ cup skimmed milk or unsweetened almond milk

Juice and zest of 1 orange

¼ teaspoon ground cinnamon

8 slices multigrain bread

Maple syrup, for serving

Directions:

Preheat the oven to 400°F. Cover a baking sheet with parchment paper and lightly spray it with cooking spray. Set aside. In a medium bowl, whisk together the eggs, milk, orange juice, orange zest, and cinnamon until well blended. Lightly dredge each bread slice in the egg mixture and shake off any excess liquid. Place the slices side by side on the baking sheet and very lightly spray the tops with cooking spray. Bake until the bread is golden brown, then turn over each slice to brown, about 12 minutes. Add a drizzle of maple syrup before serving. Nutrition:

Calories: 213

Total fat: 6g

Saturated fat: 2g

Sodium: 187mg

Carbohydrates: 27g

Fiber: 5g

Protein: 13g

4. Almond "McGriddle" Casserole

Preparation Time: 10 minutes

Cooking Time: 20 minutes

Servings: 8

Ingredients:

1-pound Breakfast sausage

.25 cup Flaxseed meal

1 cup Almond flour

10 Large eggs

6 tablespoon Maple syrup

4 ounces of cheese

4 tablespoon Butter

.5 teaspoon Onion

.5 teaspoon Garlic powder

.25 teaspoon Sage

Also Needed: 9 x 9-inch casserole dish

Directions:

Warm up the oven temperature to reach 350º Fahrenheit. Prepare the casserole dish with a sheet of parchment paper. Use the medium heat setting on the stovetop to cook the sausage in a skillet. Add all of the dry ingredients (the cheese also), and stir in the wet ones. Add 4 tablespoons of syrup. Stir and blend well. After the sausage is browned, combine all of the fixings with the grease.

Empty the mix into the casserole dish and drizzle the rest of the syrup on top. Set the timer for 45 to 55 minutes. Transfer to the countertop until it's room temperature. The casserole should be easy to remove by using the edge of the parchment paper. After the casserole has cooled; just slice it into 8 portions.

Nutrition:

Calories: 448

Protein: 26g

Fat Content: 36g

Total Net Carbs: 3 g

5. Choco Chip Whey Waffles

Preparation Time: 10 minutes

Cooking Time: 6 minutes

Servings: 2

Ingredients:

2 tablespoons organic coconut oil

2 tablespoons coconut sugar

4 tablespoons chocolate whey protein powder

⅓ cup almond flour

A pinch of salt

½ teaspoon baking powder

½ cup almond milk

2 piece eggs

Directions:

Mix all the ingredients in the blender to obtain a homogenous paste. Preheat your waffle iron. Pour the waffle dough into the iron and cook each waffle for 3 minutes.

Nutrition:

Calories: 423

Fat: 32.8g

Protein: 26.5g

Total Carbohydrates: 8.3g

Dietary Fiber: 2.9g

Net Carbohydrates: 5.4g

6. Creamy Cinnamon Scrambled Egg

Preparation Time: 10 minutes

Cooking Time: 5 minutes

Servings: 2

Ingredients:

4 eggs

1/4 teaspoon ground cinnamon

2 tablespoons heavy cream

1 tablespoon butter

Pepper

Salt

Directions:

Combine eggs and heavy cream in a bowl. Melt butter in a pan over medium heat. Add the egg mixture to a pan and stir until the eggs are cooked. Remove the pan from heat. Sprinkle it with ground cinnamon. Serve and enjoy.

Nutrition:

Calories: 186

Fat: 15 g

Carbohydrates: 1 g

Sugar: 1 g

Protein: 12 g

Cholesterol: 346 mg

7. Basil and Cherry Tomato Breakfast

Preparation Time: 4 minutes

Cooking Time: 4 hours

Servings: 4

Ingredients:

1 tablespoon olive oil

2 yellow onions, chopped

2 pounds cherry tomatoes, halved

3 tablespoons tomato puree

2 garlic cloves, minced

A pinch of sea salt and black pepper

1 bunch basil, chopped

Directions:

Cook everything in the slow cooker for 4 hours on high after greasing it with oil and adding all the ingredients. For breakfast, stir the mixture, portion it out into dishes, and serve.

Nutrition:

Calories: 90

Fat: 1g

Protein: 1g

Carbs: 1.8g"

8. Burrito Breakfast

Preparation Time: 5 minutes

Cooking Time: 10 minutes

Servings: 4

Ingredients:

4 ounces breakfast sausage

4 eggs

½ cup of grated cheddar cheese

½ cup chopped soft spinach

1/3 cup diced onion

1/3 cup diced bell pepper

A spoonful of olive oil

1.5 cups almond flour

3 tablespoons psyllium peeling powder

1/2 teaspoon baking powder

1/8 teaspoon of salt

2 proteins

4 tablespoons of boiling water

2 tablespoons deep-fry avocado oil

Directions:

FOR TORTILLA: Mix all tortilla ingredients in a small bowl; mix well. Pour boiling water into the dough and mix with a spatula. After all, components have been mixed, allow the mixture to stand for 15 minutes. Divide the dough into four equal parts. Roll each portion into a ball and create a circle of 1/8 inch between two pieces of parchment paper. Heat a large 10-inch pan over medium heat, and lightly coat the pan with avocado/olive oil. Place the omelets in the pan and bake for 30 to 60 seconds on each side until golden brown. Turn and repeat on the other side. Repeat with the remaining cakes.

FOR FILLING: Heat half of the oil in a frying pan over medium heat. Add onions and fry for a minute or two. Add pepper and sausage, cook until the sausage is well cooked. Remove fire and add spinach; Stir and let cool. Divide the remaining oil into two pans. Put both on medium heat. Stir the beaten egg into the pan until it is evenly distributed. When the egg starts laying, turn it again to place the egg evenly around the pan. When it is almost done, carefully turn the egg into the most giant pan and sprinkle it evenly with cheese on it. Prepare only a minute and slide on the plate. This is your tortilla! Place each of the four egg cookies on separate plates or together in a bowl. Place a quarter of the sausage mixture on one side of each egg and a double tortilla. Serve warm.

Nutrition:

Calories: 44.39 g

Fat 14.05g

Fiber: 7.87 g

Protein: 25.22 g

9. Chili Tomatoes and Eggs

Preparation Time: 10 minutes

Cooking Time: 20 minutes

Servings: 4

Ingredients:

1 tablespoon ghee, melted

2 shallots, chopped

2 chili peppers, minced

Salt and black pepper to taste

4 tomatoes, cubed

4 eggs, whisked

1 teaspoon sweet paprika

1 tablespoon chives, chopped

Directions:

Shallots and chili peppers should be added to a heated pan with ghee and sautéed for 5 minutes. Add the tomatoes and the other ingredients except for the eggs, toss then cook everything for 5 minutes more. Toss in the eggs, simmer the mixture for an additional five minutes, then divide it among plates and serve.

Nutrition:

Calories: 119

Fat: 7.9

Fiber: 1.8

Carbs: 6.5

Protein 6.9

10. Keto Granola Cereal

Preparation time: 30 minutes

Cooking time: 0 minutes

Servings: 3

Ingredients:

1 cup of flaxseeds

1 large egg

1 cup Almonds

1 cup Hazelnuts

1 cup Pecans

1/3 cup Pumpkin seeds

1/3 cup Sunflower seeds

1/4 cup melted butter or coconut oil or ghee   for dairy-free

1 tsp Vanilla extract

Directions:

Preheat the oven to 370 degrees F, and line the baking trays with wax or parchment paper. Chop the hazelnuts, almonds, and pecans into large pieces in a food processor by pulsing them intermittently until they are all chopped. Being softer, pecans are added later. Pulse just long enough to combine everything after adding the flaxseeds, sunflower seeds, and pumpkin seeds. Don't over-process; you should have most seeds in intact form. Whisk an egg white and pour it into the food processor.

Then, in a small bowl, combine the melted butter and vanilla essence; then, evenly pour that mixture into the food processor.

Pulse again to mix well until it combines in the form of coarse meal and nut pieces, and everything should be a little moist from the egg white and butter.

Transfer the mixture to the prepared baking tray, evenly pressing, and bake for 15 to 18 minutes, or until slightly brown from the edges. Let it cool, then break it into pieces.

Nutrition:

Calories: 441

Fat: 40g

Carbohydrates: 4g

Protein: 16g

LUNCH MEAL PLANS

Lunch

11. Satisfying Grilled Mushrooms

Preparation time: 10 minutes

Cooking time: 10 minutes

Servings: 4 minutes

Ingredients:

2 cups shiitake mushrooms

1 tablespoon balsamic vinegar

1/4 cup extra virgin olive oil

1-2 garlic cloves, minced

A handful of parsley

1 teaspoon salt

Directions:

Rinse the mushroom and pat dry; put in a foil and drizzle with balsamic vinegar and extra virgin olive oil. Sprinkle the mushroom with garlic, parsley, and salt. Grill for about 10 minutes or until tender and cooked through. Serve warm.

Nutrition:

Calories: 171

Total Fat: 12.8g

Carbs: 15.9g

Dietary Fiber: 2.4g

Protein: 1.8g

Cholesterol: 0mg

Sodium: 854m

Sugars: 4.1g

11. Simple Baked Shrimp with Béchamel Sauce

Preparation Time: 10 minutes

Cooking Time: 5-7 minutes

Servings: 4

Ingredients:

6-7 ounces shrimp

1-ounces mozzarella

4 ounces béchamel sauce (recipe provided)

1 tablespoon ghee

Directions:

Cut boiled shrimp and transfer them to a baking   dish. Pour sauce on top. Bake for 5-7 minutes. Serve and enjoy!

Nutrition:

Calories: 150

Fat: 10g

Carbohydrates: 2g

Protein: 14g

12. Cajun-Style Fish-Tomato Stew

Preparation Time: 20 minutes

Cooking Time: 35 minutes

Servings: 4

Ingredients:

1 tablespoon olive oil

1 sweet onion, chopped

1 green bell pepper, diced

3 celery stalks, sliced

1 tablespoon minced garlic

1 tablespoon Cajun seasoning

1 (15-ounce) can low-sodium diced tomatoes

1 cup low-sodium chicken broth

4 (5-ounce) boneless, skinless firm fish, cut into 1-inch pieces

1 cup shredded carrot

1 cup shredded Swiss chard

1 tablespoon chopped fresh parsley, for garnish

Directions:

In a sizable saucepan, heat the oil over medium-high heat. Sauté the onion, bell pepper, celery, and garlic until softened, about 5 minutes. Stir in the seasoning and sauté for 2 minutes more. Stir in the tomatoes and broth and bring the mixture to a boil. Medium-low heat should be used to simmer for 15 minutes. Stir in the fish and carrot and simmer until the fish is just cooked through 7 to 8 minutes. Remove from the heat, stir in the Swiss chard, and let the stew sit for 5 minutes to wilt the greens. Serve topped with parsley.

Addition Tip: This spicy creation is thick enough to be served over a cooked grain such as quinoa or brown rice. One cup of cooked brown rice will bump the calories to 427 per serving.

Nutrition:

Calories: 211

Total fat: 5g

Saturated fat: 1g

Sodium: 219 mg

Carbohydrates: 14g

Fiber: 3g

Protein: 28g

13. Asian Style Zucchini Salad

Preparation Time: 5 minutes

Cooking Time: 0 minutes

Servings: 2

Ingredient:

1.5 tablespoon Sesame oil

.5 tablespoon Almonds

1 tablespoon White vinegar

.5 cups Crumbled feta cheese

1 Medium zucchini

.5 cup Shredded cabbage

1.5 tablespoon Sunflower seeds

Directions:

Roast the almonds in a deep-frying pan using the low-temperature setting. Use a spiralizer to shred the zucchini into strips. Prepare the salad using cabbage, zucchini, almonds, and sunflower seeds. Whisk both oils and vinegar. Spritz over the salad.

Garnish with the feta and toss before serving.

Nutrition:

Calories: 846

Protein: 14 g

Fat Content: 86 g

Total Net Carbs: 7 g

14. Pulled Pepper-Lemon Loins

Preparation Time: 15 minutes

Cooking Time: 4-6 hours

Servings: 4

Ingredients:

½ stick of butter

1-piece large lemon, sliced

1-piece green pepper, chopped

1 tablespoon garlic, minced

2 tablespoons olive oil

1 tablespoon salt

1 teaspoon dried thyme

½ tablespoon Dijon mustard

3 pounds (4 pcs) chicken tenderloins

1 cheddar cheese slice, shredded

4 leaves romaine lettuce

Directions:

Combine the butter, lemon, pepper, garlic, oil, salt, thyme, and mustard in your slow cooker. Switch the slow cooker on high and melt the butter. Add the chicken; ensure to coat the chicken with the butter mixture. Cook for 4 hours on high or 6 hours on low. Add the cheese and let it sit for 15 minutes on low. To serve, place the chicken over a bed of lettuce leaves.

Nutrition:

Calories: 280

Fat: 23.3g

Protein: 14g

Total Carbohydrates: 4.1g

Dietary Fiber: 0.6g

Net Carbohydrates: 3.5g

15. Vegan Tuna Salad

Preparation Time: 5 minutes

Cooking Time: 55 minutes

Servings: 6

Ingredients:

2 cans chickpeas

1 tablespoon prepared yellow mustard

2 tablespoons vegan mayonnaise

1 tablespoon jarred capers

2 tablespoons pickle relish

½ cup chopped celery

Directions:

In a medium bowl, combine chickpeas, mustard, vegan mayo, and mustard. Pulse in a food processor or mash with a potato masher until the mixture is partially smooth with some chunks. Add the remaining ingredients to the chickpea mixture and mix until combined. Serve right away or keep chilled until you're ready to.

Nutrition:

Calories: 170

Fat: 18g

Protein: 15g

Carbs: 1.8g

16. Thai Inspired Pineapple and Chicken Salad

Preparation Time: 10 minutes

Cooking Time: 15 minutes

Serving: 2

Ingredients:

1 pinch of salt

1 pinch of ground, black pepper

2 tablespoons of white wine vinegar

1 tablespoon of chili sauce

5 oz. of cooked chicken breast, store-bought,   flavors include barbeque and lemon and herb

8 oz. of canned pineapple, finely diced

1 red onion, finely diced

1 chili, deseeded and finely sliced

3 oz. of mixed lettuce leaves

1 cup of cherry tomatoes

A handful of fresh Cilantro

Directions:

Drain the canned pineapple and retain the juice. In a large salad bowl, combine slithers of cooked chicken, diced pineapple, onion, lettuce, cherry tomatoes, and cilantro. In a separate bowl, combine the salt, pepper, vinegar, chili sauce, diced chili, and 2 tablespoons of the retained pineapple juice. Whisk together. Serve the salad with the sauce drizzled over it.

Nutrition:

Calories: 176

17. Tikka of Mushrooms and Onion

Preparation Time: 30 minutes

Cooking Time: 45 minutes

Servings: 4

Ingredients:

2/3 cup thick whipped cream

1/3 teaspoon of cumin powder

2-1/2 tablespoons lemon juice

2-1/2 teaspoons of olive oil

3/4 teaspoon of ginger and garlic paste

Salt to taste

14 small mushrooms

2/3 onions, petals

4 teaspoons of olive oil, for baking

Wooden sticks

Directions:

Take the first six ingredients in a large bowl, and mix well to make a homogeneous mixture. Add mushrooms and onions to this mixture and cover carefully. For one hour, cover and marinate in the refrigerator. Preheat the oven to 425. Put mushrooms and onions on wooden skewers. Place in the oven on a baking sheet or a baking tray for about 30 minutes, turning every 10 minutes to get a uniform preparation to guarantee. Also, grill the grill over medium heat and keep turning everywhere. Sprinkle it with lemon juice to taste and serve immediately.

Nutrition:

Calories 15.1 g

Fat 4.19 g

Total carbohydrates 1.23g

Fiber: 0.7g

Protein: 1.71g

18. Broccoli Cream

Preparation Time: 10 minutes

Cooking Time: 20 minutes

Servings: 4

Ingredients:

1-pound broccoli florets

4 cups vegetable stock

2 shallots, chopped

1 teaspoon chili powder

A pinch of salt and black pepper

2 garlic cloves, minced

2 tablespoons olive oil, chopped

1 tablespoon dill, chopped

Directions:

Heat a pot with the oil over medium-high heat; add the shallots and the garlic and sauté for 2 minutes. Add the broccoli and the other ingredients to a simmer then cook over medium heat for 18 minutes. Blend the mix using an immersion blender, divide the cream into bowls, and serve.

Nutrition:

Calories: 111

Fat: 8

Carbs: 10.2

Protein: 3.7

19. Coconut Lobster Tails

Preparation Time: 10 minutes

Cooking Time: 10 minutes

Servings: 2

Ingredients:

2 big whole lobster tails

½ teaspoon paprika

½ cup coconut butter

White pepper to the taste

1 lemon cut into wedges

Directions:

Place lobster tails on a baking sheet cut the top side of lobster shells and pull them apart. Season with white pepper and paprika. Add butter and toss gently. Introduce lobster tails in a preheated broiler and broil for 10 minutes. Divide on plates, garnish with lemon wedges, and serve right away!

Nutrition:

Calories 140g

Fat: 2g

Fiber: 2g

Carbs: 6g

Protein: 6g

20. Chicken Avocado Salad

Preparation Time: 40 minutes

Cooking Time: 20 minutes

Servings: 4

Ingredients:

1 pound of boneless chicken thighs

4 tablespoons of extra virgin olive oil

3 tablespoons of chopped celeries

2 tablespoons of cilantro

1 large ripe avocado

1 ½ teaspoons of oregano

1 tablespoon of lemon juice

½ cup almond milk ½ cup diced onion

½ teaspoon pepper

Directions:

Pour in almond milk in a bowl, add in the oregano, then stir well. The almond milk mixture should be applied to the cut-up boneless chicken thighs. Wait 13 to 15 minutes before using. Preheat an oven to 300°F, and line the baking tray with a foil sheet. Bake the coated chicken slices for 30 to 40 minutes after placing them on the baking pan. Meanwhile, slice the avocado into cubes, then drizzle some olive oil and lemon juice, and set aside. In a salad bowl, mix in the cilantro, chopped celery, and onion, and sprinkle some pepper, mix well. Take out the chicken and garnish with the avocado mix and salad. Serve warm.

Nutrition:

Calories: 256g

Total Fat: 49g

Total Carbs: 8g

Protein: 9g

DINNER MEAL PLANS

Dinner

21. Lean Steak with Oregano-Orange Chimichurri & Arugula Salad

Preparation time: 5 minutes

Cooking time: 5 minutes

Servings: 4

Ingredients:

1 teaspoon finely grated orange zest

1 teaspoon dried oregano

1 small garlic clove, grated

2 teaspoon vinegar (red wine, cider, or white wine)

1 tablespoon fresh orange juice

1/2 cup chopped fresh flat-leaf parsley leaves

1 1/2-pound lean steak, cut into 4 pieces

Sea salt and pepper

1/4 cup and 2 teaspoons extra virgin olive oil

4 cups arugula

2 bulbs of fennel, shaved

2 tablespoons whole-grain mustard

Directions:

Make chimichurri: In a medium bowl, combine orange zest, oregano, and garlic. Mix in vinegar, orange juice, and parsley, and then slowly whisk in ¼ cup of olive oil until emulsified. Season it with sea salt and pepper. Sprinkle the steak with salt and pepper; heat the remaining olive oil in a large skillet and cook the steak over medium-high heat for about 6 minutes per side or until browned. Allow to cool for at least 10 minutes after removing from heat. Add mustard to a medium bowl with the meat, greens, and fennel. Add salt and pepper to taste. Serve steak with chimichurri and salad. Enjoy!

Nutrition:

Calories: 343

Total Fat: 20.6 g

Carbs: 2 g

Dietary Fiber: 0.5 g

Sugars: 0.8 g

Protein: 0.6 g"

22. Delicious Turkey Wrap

Preparation Time: 10 minutes

Cooking Time: 10 minutes

Servings: 6

Ingredients:

1 ¼ pound of ground turkey, lean

4 green onions, minced

1 tablespoon of olive oil

1 garlic clove, minced

2 teaspoons of chili paste

8-ounce water chestnut, diced

3 tablespoons of hoisin sauce

2 tablespoons of coconut aminos

1 tablespoon of rice vinegar

12 butter lettuce leaves

1/8 teaspoon of salt

Directions:

Take a pan and place it over medium heat, add turkey and garlic to the pan. Heat it for 6 minutes until cooked. Take a bowl, and put the turkey inside. Add water chestnuts and onions. Add the vinegar, chili paste, coconut aminos, and hoisin sauce after stirring. Stir thoroughly before adding the mixture to the lettuce leaves. Serve and enjoy!

Nutrition:

Calories: 162

Fat: 4g

Net Carbohydrates: 7g

Protein: 23g

23. Pork Tenderloin Medallions with Herb Sauce

Preparation Time: 15 minutes

Cooking Time: 17 minutes

Servings: 4

Ingredients:

½ cup almond flour

Pinch sea salt

Pinch freshly ground black pepper

1-pound pork tenderloin, cut into 3-inch-thick pieces, pounded to ½-inch-thick medallions

2 tablespoons olive oil

½ cup low-sodium chicken stock

Juice and zest of 1 lemon

1 teaspoon chopped fresh parsley

1 teaspoon chopped fresh thyme

Directions:

In a small bowl, combine the almond flour, salt, and pepper. Dredge the pork medallions in the almond flour mixture and set aside. Over medium-high heat, heat the oil in a large skillet. Add the pork and pan fry until browned and cooked through, about 12 minutes, turning once. Remove the pork to a plate, cover with foil, and set aside. Add the chicken stock to the skillet, stirring to scrape up any meaty bits, and simmer until the liquid is reduced by half, about 5 minutes. Stir in the lemon juice, zest, parsley, and thyme. Add the pork back to the skillet, turning to coat the pork in the sauce, and serve warm.

Nutrition:

Calories: 226

Total fat: 14g

Carbohydrates: 2g

Fiber: 1g

Protein: 23g

24. Baked Whole Turkey

Preparation Time: 40 minutes

Cooking Time: 200 minutes

Servings: 10

Ingredient:

4 tablespoons Olive oil

10 pounds' Turkey

2 teaspoons Garlic powder

2 teaspoons Salt

1 teaspoon Thyme

1 teaspoon Paprika

1 teaspoon Pepper

5 cups of reduced-sodium chicken broth

Directions:

Rinse and pat dry the turkey, removing the giblets. Grease a roasting pan and set the oven temperature to 325° Fahrenheit. The seasonings and oil are rubbed onto the turkey. Add the liquid to the pan and arrange the turkey on top. (Internal temperature should be 165 degrees Fahrenheit.) Bake for three hours. To avoid drying out, baste roughly every hour. Let the turkey stand for about 30 minutes before slicing to serve. Add a little rosemary, or add a bit more thyme for a taste change.

Nutrition:

Calories: 39

Protein:42 g

Fat Content: 23g

Total Net Carbs: 1g

25. Shrimp with Zucchini Noodles

Preparation Time: 10 minutes

Cooking Time: 10 minutes

Servings: 6

Ingredients:

½ pound shrimp

1 tablespoon olive oil

4 zucchinis, spiralized

¼ cup + 2 tablespoons Thai sweet chili sauce

¼ cup + 2 tablespoons light mayo

¼ cup + 2 tablespoons plain Greek yogurt

1 ½ teaspoon sriracha sauce

1 ½ tablespoon honey

2 teaspoons lime juice

Direction:

Cook the shrimp till opaque. When the oil in the pan is hot, add the zucchini and cook until fork-tender. Drain it and give it ten minutes to rest. Mix all sauce components until smooth. Split up the sauce into the containers. Add the zucchini noodles and gently stir to coat well. Add the shrimp to the containers.

Nutrition:

Calories: 119

Sugar: 1g

Carbs: 4g

Total Fat: 8g

Protein: 14g

26. Pizza Pie with Cheesy Cauliflower Crust

Preparation Time: 5 minutes

Cooking time: 30 minutes

Servings: 2

Ingredients:

½ head cauliflower, rinsed, riced, cooked for 5 minutes in boiling water, and drained

2 piece eggs, whisked

⅓ parmesan cheese

½ cup cherry tomatoes, washed and halved

2 tablespoons organic hempseed oil

1 teaspoon balsamic vinegar

1 mozzarella cheese ball, crumbled

¼ cup basil leaves

Directions:

Spin the cooked cauliflower in a dish towel to let out as much liquid as possible. (The goal is to obtain a flour texture.) Add the eggs and cheese. Mix well. Spread to a disk the cauliflower dough on a baking pan lined with parchment paper. Bake for 15 minutes at 400°F in your preheated oven. Meanwhile, mix the tomatoes with hemp seed oil and balsamic vinegar. Season the mixture with salt and pepper. Remove the pizza dough from the oven. Add the tomato mixture and sprinkle over with mozzarella. Return the pan to the oven and bake further for 15 minutes. Serve hot and garnish with fresh basil leaves.

Nutrition:

Calories: 384

Fat: 32.1g

Protein: 19.9g

Total Carbohydrates: 5.5g

Carbohydrates: 3.8g

27. Coated Cauliflower Head

Preparation Time: 10 minutes

Cooking Time: 40 minutes

Servings: 6

Ingredients:

2 pounds cauliflower head

3 tablespoons olive oil

1 tablespoon butter, softened

1 teaspoon ground coriander

1 teaspoon salt

1 egg, whisked

1 teaspoon dried cilantro

1 teaspoon dried oregano

1 teaspoon tahini paste

Directions:

Trim cauliflower head if needed. Preheat the oven to 350 F. Olive oil, softened butter, salt, crushed coriander, whisked egg, dried cilantro, dried oregano, and tahini paste should all be combined in a mixing dish. Then liberally brush this mixture over the cauliflower head before placing it in the tray. For 40 minutes, bake the cauliflower head. Every 10 minutes, brush it with the remaining oil mixture.

Nutrition:

Calories: 130

Fat: 10g

Carbs: 10g

Protein: 2g

28. Mushroom Meat Creamy

Preparation Time: 5 minutes

Cooking Time: 30 minutes

Servings: 4

Ingredients:

4 tenderloin

3 tablespoons peanut butter

1 tablespoon olive oil

1 teaspoon garlic, finely chopped

1 pound of milk thistle

Salt and ground pepper to taste

1/4 cup low-sodium chicken broth

1/2 cup thick cream

chopped fresh parsley to decorate

Directions:

Add olive oil to a 10-inch cast-iron skillet that is already hot. Once the olive oil is hot, add the tenderloin and cook for 10-15 minutes until done, if desired. Place the meat on a plate and reserve. Add peanut butter to the same pan used for meat. Once the peanut butter has melted, add the garlic and leave it on the fire for 2 minutes. Add mushrooms, cook for 3-4 minutes over medium heat. Season with salt and pepper and mix well. Add chicken broth and whipped cream and cook for 4-5 minutes. Pour the sauce and cooked mushrooms over the meat. Serve hot.

Nutrition:

Calories: 388

Fat: 24.67g

Carbohydrates 9.8g

Pure Carbohydrates: 3.87g

Fiber: 3.3g

Protein: 33.38g

29. Walnut Salmon Mix

Preparation Time: 10 minutes

Cooking Time: 14 minutes

Servings: 4

Ingredients:

4 salmon filets, boneless

2 tablespoons avocado oil

A pinch of salt and black pepper

1 tablespoon lime juice

2 shallots, chopped

2 tablespoons walnuts, chopped

2 tablespoons parsley, chopped

Directions:

Heat the oil in a pan over medium-high heat; add the shallots, swirl, and cook for 2 minutes. Cook the fish and the other ingredients for 6 minutes on each side, then divide among plates and serve.

Nutrition:

Calories: 276

Fat: 14.2

Carbs: 2.7

Protein: 35.8

30. White Steamed Fish

Preparation Time: 10 minutes

Cooking Time: 10 minutes

Servings: 4

Ingredients:

4 white fish filets

1 tablespoon olive oil

1 teaspoon thyme, dried

1-pound cherry tomatoes, halved

1 cup black olives, pitted and chopped, soaked for 5 hours

A pinch of sea salt and black pepper

1 garlic clove, minced

1 cup water

Directions:

Put the water in your instant pot, place the steamer basket on top, and arrange the fish inside. Season it with salt, thyme, pepper, and garlic. Add oil, olives, and tomatoes, rub gently, cover your instant pot, and cook on Low for 10 minutes. Release the pressure fast, divide fish and all veggies between plates, and serve hot.

Nutrition:

Calories 140

Fat: 2

Fiber: 2

Carbs: 8

Protein: 2

31. Baked Lamb Ribs Macadamia with Tomato Salsa

Preparation time: 40 minutes

Cooking time: 50 minutes

Servings: 2

Ingredients:

½ pound of fresh lamb ribs

½ cup of cherry tomatoes

½ teaspoon pepper

½ cup of macadamia

½ tablespoon of macadamia oil

¼ cup fresh parsley

1 teaspoon of balsamic vinegar

1 teaspoon of minced garlic

2 tablespoons of extra virgin olive oil

Directions:

Cut lamb ribs into strips or pieces. Preheat the oven to 210°C, and line the baking tray with aluminum foil. Place the macadamia, garlic, parsley, pepper, and olive oil, in the food processor. Blend till the mixture is smooth and lump-free. Rub your processed mixture all over the lamb pieces, and coat well enough. Arrange your strips nicely in the baking tray and bake for 20-25 minutes. Meanwhile, slice the cherry tomatoes into ¼ pieces, then place them in an aluminum cup. Pour macadamia oil on the tomatoes. Use a spoon to mix the oil and tomatoes without squishing them. The aim is to get the oil all over it. Take out the cooked lamb on a plate. Place your tomatoes in the oven for 4-5 minutes, take out, and drizzle with balsamic vinegar, stir well. Pour the tomatoes on the lamb and serve warm.

Nutrition:

Calories: 241

Total Fat: 22.1g

Total Carbs: 1.5g

Protein: 10.1g

Here are some ways for dealing with hunger and cravings throughout your fasting periods:

Choose the best intermittent fasting method:

Different intermittent fasting methods suit different people. Experiment with various fasting windows and schedules to find the one that works best for you. The 16/8 approach, alternate-day fasting, and the 5:2 diet are all common methods. Finding the correct strategy can assist in reducing hunger and cravings.

Stay hydrated: Drinking enough water throughout the day can help keep hunger at bay. We frequently confuse thirst for hunger, so drink water, herbal tea, or other non-caloric liquids to stay hydrated. Drink at least 8 cups (64 ounces) of water every day, and more if necessary.

Eat nutrient-dense meals: When it's time to break your fast, emphasize nutrient-dense foods that include critical vitamins, minerals, and fiber. Include a variety of lean proteins, healthy fats, and complex carbohydrates in your meals. These macronutrients help you feel fuller for longer and prevent cravings.

Increase your fiber intake: Fiber-rich foods such as vegetables, fruits, legumes, and whole grains can help you feel full and content. They take longer to digest, enabling a continuous flow of energy and minimizing cravings. Aim for 25-30 grams of fiber every day.

Choose protein-rich foods: Including protein in your meals is critical for controlling hunger. Protein takes longer to digest and aids in the regulation of hunger hormones. To help you stay full and prevent cravings, include lean meats, fish, eggs, dairy products, lentils, and plant-based protein sources in your meals.

Practice mindful eating: Slow down and pay attention to your food when eating mindfully. Chew your food fully and taste it. Mindful eating makes you more aware of your body's hunger and fullness signals, which helps you avoid overeating within your meal window.

Keep yourself occupied and distracted: Keeping yourself active and engaged in activities can take your attention off eating cravings. Distract yourself by engaging in hobbies, exercising, reading a book, or spending time with friends and family.

Use Natural appetite suppressants :
suppressants such as green tea, black coffee, and herbal teas can help reduce hunger and cravings. To keep the calorie count low, limit your caffeine intake and avoid adding sugar or creamers to your beverages.

Get enough sleep: Sleep deprivation can boost appetite and cravings. Make sure you receive enough sleep to support your overall health and appetite. Each night, aim for 7-9 hours of quality sleep.

Control your stress: Stress can cause emotional eating and desires for harmful foods. To assist relieve stress, try stress-reduction practices like meditation, deep breathing exercises, yoga, or regular physical activity.

It's common to feel hungry and crave certain foods while fasting, especially at first. These sensations normally fade as your body adjusts to the fasting schedule. It is critical to listen to your body, eat healthy foods, and figure out what works best for you. If you have any concerns or special dietary requirements, you should seek the advice of a healthcare expert or a trained dietician.

FAQs (Frequently Asked Questions)

Is it safe for middle-aged women to fast intermittently?

Intermittent fasting is healthy for middle-aged women, but proceed with caution and speak with a healthcare expert before making any significant changes to your diet or lifestyle. Overall health, any pre-existing medical issues, and medications should all be considered. It's also critical to pay attention to your body and adapt your fasting schedule accordingly. A healthcare practitioner can offer personalized advice and help you determine whether intermittent fasting is safe and appropriate for you.

How long should fasting and eating periods last?

Depending on personal preferences and health considerations, intermittent fasting might have different fasting and eating periods. Two popular methods are:

1. The 16/8 method: This calls for a 16-hour fast followed by an 8-hour eating window each day. You can decide to eat between 12:00 and 8:00 p.m. and observe a fast from 8:00 p.m. to 12:00 p.m. the following day.

2. The 5:2 approach, in which you eat normally five days a week and limit calories to 500–600 for two separate days, is another option.

Can I drink water or other beverages while fasting?

Yes, water and other non-caloric drinks like black tea or plain tea are often OK during intermittent fasting. It's crucial to stay hydrated, and drinking these beverages can help you do that when you're fasting. The benefits of fasting can be hampered if you add sugar, cream, or any other calorie-containing additives to your drinks, which is why it's crucial to avoid doing so. Any beverages you take while fasting should be considered in terms of their total calorie count.

What am I allowed to eat during the eating window?

You are free to eat your typical meals and foods throughout the intermittent fasting eating window. Although there are no particular restrictions on the kinds of food you can eat, it is generally advised to concentrate on wholesome, nutritional foods to promote your general health. Various fruits, vegetables, lean proteins, whole grains, and healthy fats are included in this.

Should I use vitamins while fasting intermittently?

As long as you are maintaining a balanced and nutritious diet within your eating window, additional vitamin supplements are typically not required if you are using intermittent fasting. Your body needs a variety of vital vitamins and minerals, which are included in whole meals. It's crucial to speak with a healthcare provider or a qualified dietitian, though, if you have particular nutritional deficits or medical conditions that call for vitamin supplementation. They can determine your specific needs, advise you on whether supplements are required, and show you how to successfully include them in your fasting practice.

Will Intermittent Fasting Cause Muscle Loss?

One of the most common fears with intermittent fasting is that you will lose lean muscle mass. Many people believe that if you skip a meal, your body will immediately begin burning off the protein in your muscles as an energy source, but this is not the case, owing to human evolution. You cannot live without energy, so even if you do not eat, your body will find a method to obtain it. Its preferred fuel is glucose, which can be obtained from carbs or glycogen stored in your liver or muscles. Its second preferred source is your body fat, which is effectively surplus energy stored for later use.

As long as you consume enough calories, your body understands that it should not use muscle as its major energy source and will only use it as a last resort when glucose is depleted and body fat is insufficient to support life. This occurs at roughly 4% body fat, which is exceedingly low. Female athletes, on the other hand, often have 1420 percent body fat. So, unless you get below 4% body fat, your body will do everything it can to preserve lean muscle mass. Excessive calorie restriction can indeed induce muscle loss while also slowing your metabolism. But keep in mind: Intermittent fasting is not the same as calorie restriction.

Fasting has been shown in studies to help enhance lean muscle mass and grow muscle rather than break it down. Fasting causes your body to create more human growth hormone and testosterone, which improves insulin sensitivity. This combination of actions aids in muscle building and recovery after exercise.

Is it safe for women with thyroid problems to fast?

Women with thyroid disorders are often advised not to fast, but it is not fasting itself that poses a risk. It's a matter of calories. T4, the inactive thyroid hormone, increases and competes with T3, the active thyroid hormone, when calories are restricted. This can result in a 50% drop in active T3, which can aggravate pre-existing hypothyroidism.

Even if you have hypothyroidism, there is evidence that fasting can help reduce your dependency on thyroid medication and improve fasting insulin and insulin resistance. If you have a thyroid problem, consult your doctor first, and then do the following: Begin slowly. Begin with shorter fasting protocols, such as 12/12, and work your way up to 14/8 if you feel comfortable. Pay close attention to what you eat. Reduce your intake of sugar, which can feed the nasty bacteria in your gut, as well as gluten and dairy, which can cause inflammation and exacerbate pre-existing thyroid disorders. Don't limit your calories by more than 20%. If you require 2,000 calories per day to maintain your weight, don't consume less than 1,600.

Don't overwork yourself. Working out too hard might have a bad impact on your thyroid, especially if you're fasting. Keep exercises light, at least at first. If necessary, take vitamins. Selenium, iodine, zinc, and omega-3 fatty acids are essential for anyone suffering from thyroid problems.NSAIDs should be avoided to the greatest extent possible. NSAIDs, such as aspirin and ibuprofen, can reduce thyroid hormone levels by preventing T4 and T3 from attaching to carrier proteins. If you must take NSAIDs, do so with a meal.

Can Fasting Cause Eating Disorders?

Many women have expressed concern about fasting causing an eating disorder or binge-eating behavior.

There is evidence that protracted periods of intense calorie restriction can raise the risk of future food binges. But keep two things in mind: Intermittent fasting is not the same as calorie restriction. It is recommended that you consume all of the calories you require when fasting intermittently. While long periods of calorie restriction may be connected with binge-eating behaviors, shorter periods of calorie restriction did not have the same effect. There is no evidence that a properly designed, nutrient-rich intermittent fasting strategy will initiate an eating disorder or make binge eating more probable in healthy women without a history of eating disorders.

The temptation to binge is frequently triggered by the substantial dips and surges in blood sugar that occur following a carbohydrate-rich meal. After a while of intermittent fasting, your blood sugar levels tend to stabilize and you have less of an urge to overeat. If you have a history of disordered eating or are prone to obsessive and/or compulsive behavior around food, you should avoid any type of dietary restriction, including intermittent fasting. Seek the assistance of a health expert if you are concerned about yourself or notice any unusual eating patterns or behaviors.

Why am I nauseous in the morning if I don't eat?

Feeling sick in the morning indicates that your circadian rhythms are out of sync. If you didn't get enough sleep or if you tossed and turned all night, it can mess with your hormones and make you feel ill. It's also conceivable that anything you're consuming is causing you discomfort. This is especially more likely if you've made considerable dietary adjustments in addition to incorporating intermittent fasting. If you've been intermittent fasting for several weeks and you're still feeling unwell in the morning, try the following: Examine your sleeping habits. Are you getting enough uninterrupted sleep and going to bed early enough? If not, examine your sleeping environment and make the required modifications to improve your sleep.

Do you go to bed and get up at the same time every day?

Consider what you're eating. Is there anything that causes digestive discomfort, bloating, or heartburn? Anything that you aren't processing properly can cause nausea. Pay attention to any meals that seem to upset you regularly, and then try to avoid them for a few weeks to see if it helps. Examine your stress levels. Even if you aren't aware that you are stressed or anxious, stress and worry can cause nausea. Outside of fasting, make sure you're keeping a self-care regimen and managing your stress.

Can I Fast If I Have Hormonal Issues, Such as PCOS?

Because one of the concerns of fasting is hormone disruption, you may believe that if you already have hormonal disorders, such as polycystic ovarian syndrome (PCOS), you are not a suitable candidate for intermittent fasting. However, this is not always the case. Androgen hormones, which include testosterone and androstenedione, are commonly thought of as male hormones, but women generate them as well, albeit in smaller quantities. The production of androgen hormones increases in PCOS, resulting in a hormonal imbalance known as hyperandrogenism. This higher amount of androgen hormones leads to infertility, trouble getting pregnant, and/or undesirable metabolic alterations such as insulin resistance, high insulin levels, high cholesterol and triglycerides, and weight gain. There is no one cause of PCOS, but insulin resistance and elevated insulin levels play a crucial part in the hormonal imbalance and the symptoms that accompany it. While conventional nutrition advice for PCOS recommends eating many small meals throughout the day to keep blood sugar and insulin levels stable, intermittent fasting improves insulin levels and thus insulin resistance better than constantly eating. Intermittent fasting has been shown in studies to reduce insulin growth factor 1, glucose, and insulin levels, which can improve ovarian function, decrease androgen hormones, and reduce reproductive problems in women with PCOS. This is true for all types of intermittent fasting, including alternate-day, time-restricted, 5:2, and spontaneous fasting.

Will Endometriosis Be Helped by Fasting?

There hasn't been any research that specifically studied the effects of fasting on endometriosis as of 2020, therefore there's no conclusive answer as to whether fasting can help. However, given the underlying reasons for endometriosis and fasting's effect on hormones in general, it seems reasonable to believe that fasting could help improve the condition. While there is no one cause of endometriosis, one common feature is elevated estrogen levels or estrogen dominance. As a result, medical specialists have labeled it an "estrogen-dependent" condition.

Intermittent fasting has been demonstrated to balance hormones such as estrogen and progesterone when done correctly. Intermittent fasting also improves insulin sensitivity, which may help reverse insulin resistance, which is linked to estrogen dominance and weight gain. Weight gain and obesity, it just so happens, are important risk factors for endometriosis. Stress management is particularly critical since your body depletes progesterone when it produces the stress hormone cortisol. And when progesterone levels are low, you're in an estrogen-dominant state. If you have a chronic medical condition, you should always see your doctor before making any big lifestyle changes.

Is There an Ideal Time to Fast?

There is no unique golden hour for timing your intermittent fast that will guarantee the finest outcomes. Fasting in the early evening and overnight, followed by eating later in the day, appears to have the greatest visible benefits. As the day progresses, you become more insulin resistant and your bloodstream does not remove glucose as efficiently as it did earlier in the day. People who eat earlier in the afternoon and evening have a higher blood lipid profile, and better blood sugar management, and find it easier to maintain a healthy weight than those who eat late at night, according to studies.

According to research, those who eat late at night make fewer nutritious food choices than those who eat early. When it becomes dark, that bag of chips or those French fries appear to scream out even louder. While eating dinner at 10 p.m. and then your first meal at 12 the next day legally constitutes time-restricted fasting, it's probably not the greatest schedule. To gain the best benefits, aim to have your final meal between 6 and 8 p.m.

How Long Will It Take to See Results?

Because every woman is unique, everyone will have a different answer to this question. The consensus is that you should give intermittent fasting ten to twelve weeks before deciding whether or not it works for you. However, that takes 10 to twelve weeks of regularity. That entails fully committing to the process and adhering to your intermittent fasting strategy exactly as planned. Having said that, many ladies see the effects much sooner than that. Within a few days, you should feel less bloated and burdened. As the week progresses, you may notice that you have more energy and that any brain fog and/or sluggishness is lifting. After a few weeks, you may notice improvements in your skin, and aches and pains begin to subside.

Even if you have a long-term goal, such as losing weight, try to concentrate on these tiny, steady changes in your health as you work towards your larger objective. Celebrating all of your accomplishments will make it easier to stay to your goal.

Is it permissible to fast if I work the night shift?

If you work the night shift, you probably don't need to be informed that it can be quite taxing on your body. While intermittent fasting cannot eliminate all of the potential negative consequences, it can be made to function and gain some of the benefits. If feasible, schedule your shift during your fasting window to avoid having to eat overnight. Your schedule might look like this:

Fasting window: 11p.m to 3p.m the following day (work from 11p.m to 7a.m , sleep from when you arrive home to 3 p.m.) Eating window: 3 p.m to 11 p.m This may not be suitable if you work longer night shifts. Instead of eating late at night, you could consider eating in the morning hours of your shift. Working the night shift can alter your circadian cycle, even when fasting, so when you do eat, consume largely low-carb, high-fat items. You don't have to follow a ketogenic diet; merely a low-carb diet would suffice.

Will fasting cause my blood sugar to drop too low?

When you initially begin intermittent fasting, you may experience low blood sugar symptoms such as headache, irritability, and hunger. These symptoms can be exacerbated if you're used to eating a lot of carbohydrates and have converted to a low-carb diet plan, or if you have insulin resistance or blood sugar regulation issues. While these symptoms are unpleasant, most healthy people's blood sugar will not fall low enough to cause concern. Your body has physiological processes in place to control your blood sugar levels within a set range so you don't pass out or face other major health problems. Your body adjusts and your blood sugar is maintained even more securely as you become more sensitive to insulin and get off the blood sugar roller coaster you've been on. When this occurs, you are unlikely to experience any symptoms, including hunger, during your fasting period. This does not apply if you have diabetes. If you have type 1 diabetes, you should never fast without the consent and close supervision of your doctor. Some studies show that type 1 diabetics can reduce their insulin doses by following a fasting plan for a while, but if you don't do it correctly, or if you don't ease into it slowly and combine fasting with the right types of foods, it can lead to dangerously low blood sugar levels.

Is it normal to be constantly hungry?

There is no way to forecast how you will feel when you first begin intermittent fasting because every woman is different. If you're used to eating five or six times a day or late at night, you'll most certainly feel hungry during your fasting window during the first few weeks. You'll probably experience more acute cravings as well. This is frequently due to emotional or mental hunger rather than actual physical hunger. As your body adjusts throughout the first few weeks, your blood sugar and insulin levels begin to stabilize, and this is where the magic happens. Your appetite should subside, and you should have consistent energy throughout the day. However, if you've been following an intermittent fasting strategy for several weeks and still feel hungry, you'll need to do some troubleshooting: Calculate your calorie requirements and then track your diet for a few days to ensure you meet them. Increase your serving amounts if you're under.

Make sure you're getting enough healthy fats; they're necessary for feeling full. Avocados, olives, olive oil, grass-fed butter, ghee, fatty fish, nuts, and seeds should all be included in your diet. Examine your protein consumption. You should consume approximately 0.8-1.0

grams of protein per kilogram of body weight. Drink plenty of water. Thirst can masquerade as hunger at times.

Can I Work on Weekends?

One of the benefits of intermittent fasting is the flexibility it provides. Adjusting your fasting schedule when you have social gatherings or things you wish to accomplish on the weekend is part of that flexibility. If you're a gregarious and outgoing person and the prospect of having to fast on weekends prevents you from participating, create your fasting schedule. You can fast on Tuesday and Thursday using the 5:2 approach, or you can rotate between Tuesday, Thursday, and Saturday fasting and just fast on one weekend day. You can even fast for fourteen hours a day, seven days a week, and then relax on the weekends. Of course, the more you keep to your strategy and make wise decisions, especially on weekends, the better your outcomes will be. But intermittent fasting is designed to be a lifestyle; it can't feel like a prison sentence if you want to continue with it long-term. You must be able to balance it with your other interests.

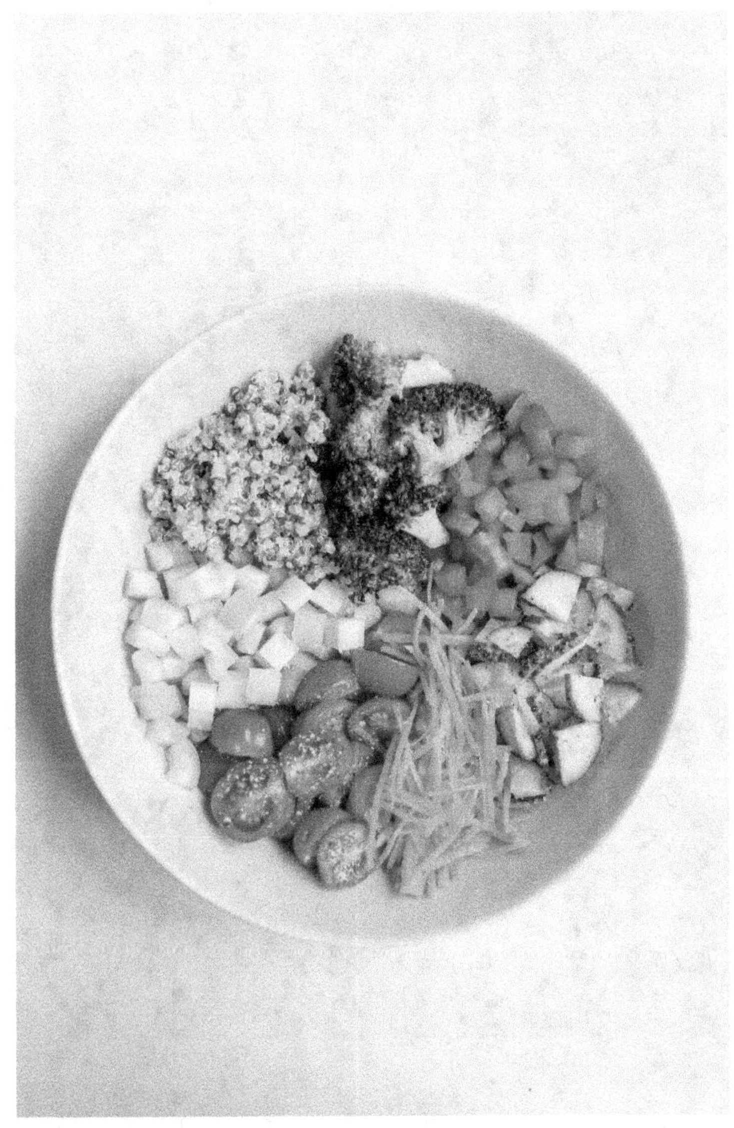

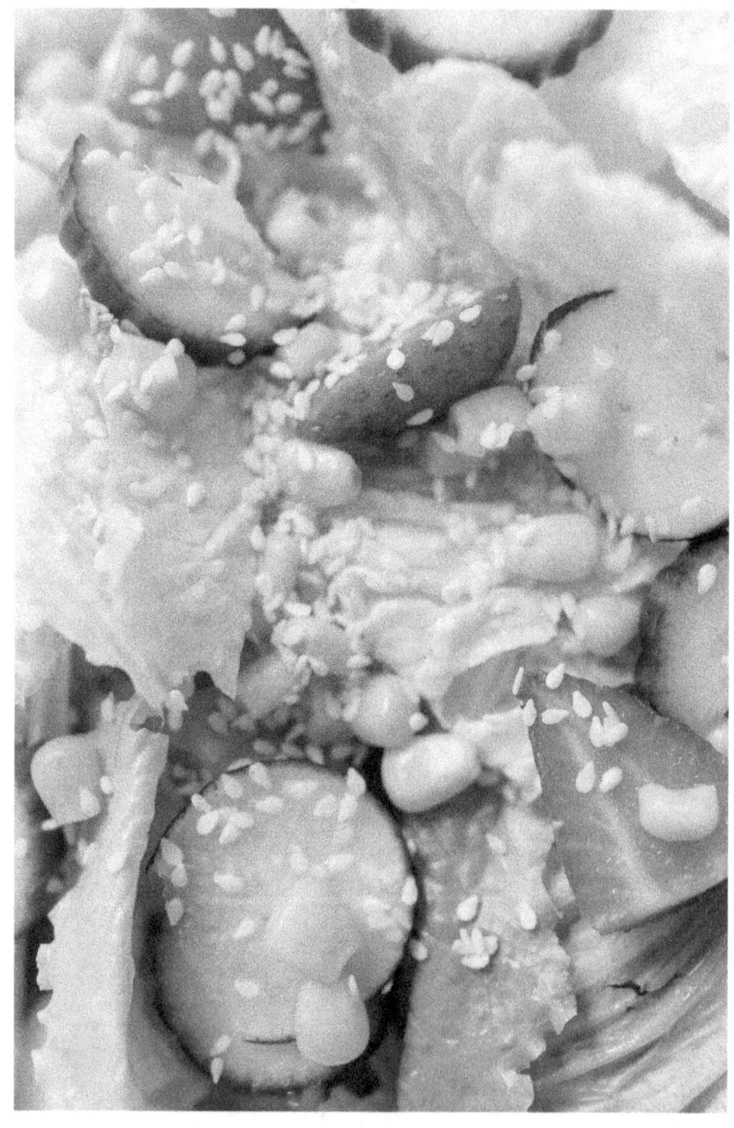

Chapter 4

Anti-inflammatory Nutrition

What is Inflammation?

Inflammation is the body's immune system's natural response to infection, injury, or tissue damage. It is a complicated process involving the release of numerous substances and immune cells that work together to combat unwanted stimuli and promote healing. Acute or chronic inflammation can occur. Acute inflammation is a short-term response to tissue damage or infection that is characterized by redness, swelling, heat, pain, and loss of function in the affected area.

Chronic inflammation, on the other hand, is a long-term response that can last weeks, months, or even years and can lead to the development of diseases such as rheumatoid arthritis, asthma, and heart disease.

While inflammation is an important aspect of the body's immunological response, persistent inflammation can be damaging and should be monitored and treated accordingly. Disease and Chronic Inflammation Middle-aged women are more likely to develop various chronic inflammatory disorders, including

Rheumatoid arthritis: This autoimmune illness causes joint inflammation, resulting in pain, stiffness, and decreased mobility. This is more common in middle-aged women than in males, and it can be especially severe for women around menopause.

Lupus: Lupus is an autoimmune condition that causes inflammation throughout the body, causing joint discomfort, exhaustion, and skin rashes. Lupus affects women nine times more than males, and it usually occurs in middle life.

Type 2 diabetes: This chronic disease is characterized by high blood sugar levels, which can cause inflammation throughout the body. Middle-aged women who are overweight or have a family history of diabetes are at a higher risk of getting type 2 diabetes.

Cardiovascular illness: Chronic inflammation can contribute to the development of heart disease, which is the leading cause of mortality among women in the United States. Middle-aged women who smoke, have high blood pressure or cholesterol or are overweight are at a higher risk of getting cardiovascular disease.

Inflammatory bowel disease: This collection of disorders, which includes Crohn's disease and ulcerative colitis, causes inflammation in the digestive tract. Women are more prone than men to acquire inflammatory bowel disease, which usually presents in young adulthood or middle age.

How Anti-Inflammatory Nutrition Can Benefit You

Anti-inflammatory nutrition can benefit middle-aged women in a variety of ways:

Reducing inflammation: As women become older, their bodies become more prone to inflammation, which can contribute to chronic health issues including heart disease, arthritis, and even some types of cancer. Anti-inflammatory foods can help reduce inflammation in the body and lower the risk of developing these illnesses.

Managing menopausal symptoms: Menopause can cause a slew of unpleasant symptoms, including hot flashes, nocturnal sweats, and mood swings. Anti-inflammatory foods including leafy greens, fatty salmon, and almonds can help alleviate these symptoms.

Improving gut health: Gut health is important for general health and well-being. Fermented meals and fiber-rich fruits and vegetables, for example, can help build healthy gut flora and enhance digestion.

Supporting good weight management: As women age, their metabolism slows, making maintaining a healthy weight more difficult.

Anti-inflammatory foods can help you lose weight by delivering the necessary nutrients and fiber that keep you full and happy. Foods that Reduce Inflammation

Fruits and Vegetables

Whole Grains

Healthy Fats

Spices and Herbs

Protein Sources

Fruits and vegetables are high in antioxidants, which aid in the battle against inflammation. Choose a variety of bright fruits and vegetables to ensure you get a variety of antioxidants. Fruits and vegetables can help with inflammation. Here are a couple of such examples:

Berries: Berries high in antioxidants and flavonoids, such as strawberries, blueberries, raspberries, and blackberries, can help reduce inflammation in the body. Berries contain a lot of antioxidants: Berries are high in antioxidants, which are substances that help protect cells from free radical damage. Free radicals can produce oxidative stress, which has been related to a variety of diseases such as cancer, heart disease, and Alzheimer's. Antioxidants can aid in the neutralization of free radicals, lowering the risk of certain diseases.

Berries can help reduce inflammation: Chronic inflammation in the body is connected to many chronic diseases, including heart disease, cancer, and diabetes. Berries include chemicals that can help reduce inflammation, lowering the chance of developing certain diseases.

Berries can help with heart health: Berries include a lot of fiber, which can help decrease cholesterol and enhance heart health. They also include flavonoids, which can enhance blood flow and lower the risk of heart disease. Berries have a low sugar content and a high fiber content, which can help manage blood sugar levels. This is critical for preventing type 2 diabetes, which is more prevalent in middle-aged women.

Berries are a nutritious and tasty addition to any diet, and they can aid in the prevention of many ailments that are common in middle-aged women. Whole grains are high in fiber, which has been demonstrated to have anti-inflammatory properties.

Reduced risk of heart disease: Whole grains contain fiber, which can help lower cholesterol and lower the risk of heart disease. Middle-aged women are at a greater risk of heart disease, and eating more whole grains can help lessen that risk.

Reduced risk of type 2 diabetes: Whole grains have a lower glycemic index than refined grains, which means they don't boost blood sugar levels as much. This can help reduce the likelihood of getting type 2 diabetes.

Reduced risk of certain cancers: Research has shown that consuming whole grains can reduce the risk of breast cancer and colon cancer. Including whole grains in your diet can be especially advantageous for middle-aged women because they have a higher chance of developing breast cancer.

Lessening the risk of obesity: Whole grains are more full than refined grains, which may lessen the likelihood of overeating and weight gain. By including whole grains in their diets, middle-aged women can reduce their risk of developing obesity, which can result in several health issues.

Lower risk of inflammation: Antioxidants and other nutrients included in whole grains may aid to lower inflammation in the body. Reducing chronic inflammation may be advantageous for middle-aged women because it has been associated with several disorders, including diabetes, cancer, and heart disease. Overall, middle-aged women can lower their chance of developing several diseases and enhance their general health by incorporating whole grains into their diet.

Nuts and seeds: It has been demonstrated that the good fats found in nuts and seeds can lower inflammation. To eliminate additional salt and oils, choose raw or unsalted nuts and seeds.

Heart Health: Nuts and seeds are an excellent source of monounsaturated and polyunsaturated fats, which can lower bad cholesterol levels (LDL) and raise levels of good cholesterol (HDL), thus lowering the risk of heart disease.

Diabetes Prevention: Because nuts and seeds have a low glycemic index, they do not induce a dramatic jump in blood sugar levels, they are a great snack for those with diabetes or pre-diabetes.

Cancer Prevention: Nuts and seeds are high in antioxidants, which assist in protecting cells and lowering the risk of cancer.

Flaxseeds, for example, contain lignans, a chemical related to a lower risk of breast cancer.

Bone health: Nuts and seeds are high in calcium, magnesium, and phosphorus, all of which are important for bone health and can help reduce the risk of osteoporosis.

Brain health: Nuts and seeds are high in vitamin E and other antioxidants, which help protect the brain from oxidative stress, which can lead to cognitive decline Incorporating a variety of nuts and seeds into your diet will assist deliver these health benefits while also combating numerous ailments in middle-aged women. However, keep in mind that nuts and seeds are high in calories, so moderation is vital. Fatty fish: Fatty fish, such as salmon, sardines, and tuna, have high levels of omega-3 fatty acids, which have anti-inflammatory properties. At least two servings of fatty fish each week are recommended.

Lower your risk of heart disease: Omega-3 fatty acids have been found to reduce inflammation, blood pressure, and triglyceride levels, all of which can contribute to a lower risk of heart disease.

Improve brain health: Omega-3 fatty acids have been linked to better cognitive function and a lower risk of Alzheimer's disease.

Prevent cancer: Omega-3 fatty acids have been demonstrated to decrease the growth of certain types of cancer cells and may have anticancer qualities.

strengthen bone health: According to research, omega-3 fatty acids may assist strengthen bone density, lowering the risk of osteoporosis in middle-aged women.

Herbs and spices: Anti-inflammatory effects are found in many herbs and spices. Ginger, turmeric, garlic, and cinnamon are a few examples.

Anti-inflammatory properties: Many herbs and spices have anti-inflammatory chemicals that can aid in the reduction of inflammation in the body. Chronic inflammation has been related to several health problems such as heart disease, diabetes, and cancer.

Antioxidant properties: Antioxidants are substances that help protect the body from oxidative stress and free radicals, both of which can cause cell damage and contribute to disease development. Herbs and spices are high in antioxidants, which can help lower the risk of developing chronic diseases.

Hormonal balancing: Some herbs and spices, such as turmeric and maca, have been demonstrated to help middle-aged women balance their hormones. Hormonal imbalances can cause a variety of health problems, such as weight gain, mood fluctuations, and decreased energy levels.

Digestive health: For centuries, several herbs and spices have been used to support digestive health. Ginger, for example, has been demonstrated to help ease nausea and aid digestion, and peppermint can assist treat digestive concerns like bloating and gas.

Support for the immune system: Herbs and spices can also aid in the immune system's defense against illnesses. For instance, it has been demonstrated that garlic contains antibacterial properties and can help prevent bacterial and viral illnesses.

Processed foods should be avoided

Foods that have been processed: Processed foods can contain a lot of salt, sugar, and bad fats. Additionally, they could include additives and preservatives that are bad for your health.

Foods high in sugar: Eating too much sugar can result in weight gain, a higher risk of diabetes, and other health issues.

Fried foods: Fried foods frequently contain high levels of calories, bad fats, and sodium, all of which raise the risk of heart disease and other illnesses.

Alcohol: Excessive alcohol consumption can result in weight gain, liver damage, and other medical issues. It may also make women more susceptible to developing breast cancer.

Red meat: Overeating red meat, especially processed red meat, has been associated with a higher risk of heart disease and a few types of cancer.

High-fat dairy: Products high in saturated fat and calories, such as cheese and butter, can raise the risk of heart disease and other illnesses.

Making an anti-inflammatory meal plan.

Tips for Meal Planning

Emphasize full, nutritious foods:

Add a lot of fruits and vegetables, whole grains, lean proteins, and healthy fats to your diet. These foods are a good source of antioxidants, vitamins, and minerals, which can aid to lessen inflammation in the body.

Choose anti-inflammatory foods: Certain foods, including fatty fish, nuts, seeds, and spices like turmeric and ginger, have natural anti-inflammatory effects. Include these foods in your meals to aid in the reduction of inflammation.

Avoid processed and sugary foods: These foods are frequently heavy in harmful fats and refined carbs, which can cause inflammation in the body. Limit your consumption of these foods as much as you can.

Include herbs and spices: Herbs and spices with anti-inflammatory effects, such as basil, oregano, rosemary, thyme, and cinnamon, can flavor your food without adding calories.

Use healthy fats when cooking: Using healthy fats when cooking, such as coconut oil, avocado oil, or olive oil, can assist to lessen inflammation in the body.

Stay hydrated: Drinking enough water throughout the day can help to wash toxins out of the body and minimize inflammation. Aim for at least 8 glasses of water per day.

Plan ahead of time: Spend some time planning out your meals and snacks for the week. This might help you stay on track and make healthy choices throughout the week. Remember that making minor modifications to your diet over time can lead to significant benefits in your general health and well-being.

Anti-Inflammatory Diet

Breakfast: Steel-cut oats with almond milk, topped with fresh berries and sliced almonds Green tea

Mid-morning snack: Apple slices with almond butter

Lunch: Grilled chicken breast with roasted sweet potatoes and sautéed kale Water with lemon slices

Snack in the afternoon: Carrots and celery sticks with hummus

Dinner: Baked salmon with quinoa and steamed broccoli Herbal tea with mixed green salad and balsamic vinaigrette Anti-Inflammatory Supplements

Probiotics Omega-3 Fatty Acids, Curcumin, Vitamin D, and Magnesium I

Lifestyle Factors that affect inflammation

Exercise, Stress Reduction, Sleep

Diet: The foods we eat can either stimulate or lessen inflammation. A diet high in sugar, saturated and trans fats, and refined carbohydrates can increase inflammation, whereas a diet rich in fruits, vegetables, whole grains, nuts, and fatty fish can lower inflammation.

Exercise: Regular physical activity can help lessen inflammation. Exercise inhibits the production of inflammatory molecules while increasing the production of anti-inflammatory molecules.

Stress: Chronic stress can result in inflammation. Cortisol and other stress hormones are released when we are under stress, and they can worsen inflammation. Deep breathing, yoga, and other relaxation exercises can help lower stress and inflammation.

Rest: Not getting enough rest might make inflammation worse. Lack of sleep can increase the production of inflammatory cytokines, but getting enough sleep can assist decrease inflammation.

Alcohol and smoking: Both smoking and binge drinking can make inflammation worse.

Environmental toxins: Exposure to environmental toxins such as pesticides, heavy metals, and air pollution can exacerbate inflammation. We can lessen inflammation in the body and enhance general health by adopting a healthy lifestyle that includes a balanced diet, consistent exercise, stress management, enough sleep, and avoiding dangerous substance

The mid-life diet for women

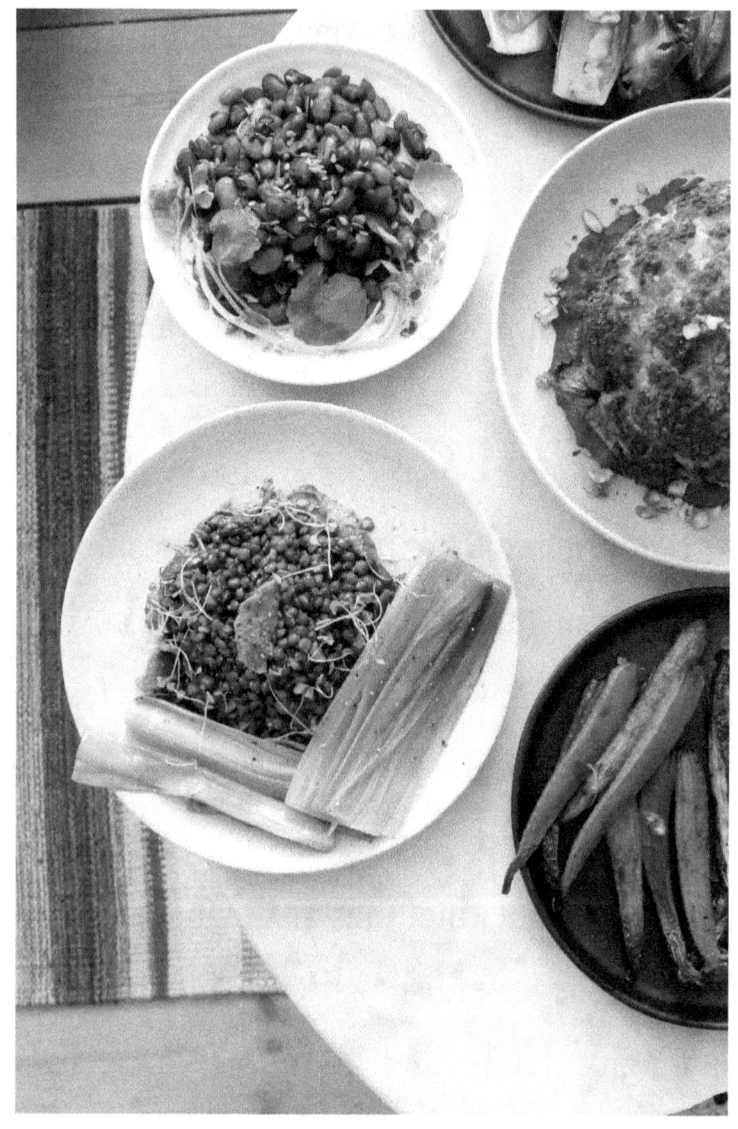

Chapter 5

Fuel Refocus

Ketosis for Fat Burning

The science behind shifting your energy usage from carbohydrates to fat

Ketosis is a metabolic state where your body switches from using carbohydrates for energy to using fat for energy. The science underlying this procedure involves your body using various fuel sources as an energy source. When you eat carbs, your body converts them to glucose, which then circulates throughout your body. After that, the glucose is sent to your cells, where it is used as fuel. Because it is accessible and simple to use, glucose is the preferred energy source for your body. However, when you limit your carbohydrate consumption, your body is compelled to find alternative energy sources. It begins to disintegrate fat stores into molecules known as ketones, which can be used as a substitute energy source.

As your body begins to use ketones for energy, your liver produces more ketones to satisfy your needs. This is known as ketogenesis. When you reach ketosis, your body becomes more efficient at burning fat for energy. It is crucial to highlight that eating a high-fat diet is not for everyone and should be undertaken with caution. Some studies, however, show that a diet rich in healthy fats may be especially advantageous for middle-aged women. High-fat diets can provide energy to middle-aged women, which is one way they can benefit. Women's metabolisms slow down as they age, which can contribute to weariness and a lack of enthusiasm to exercise.

What Exactly Are Ketones?

Ketones have recently risen to prominence as a result of the growing popularity of the ketogenic, or keto, diet, but people have relied on ketones as a source of energy for hundreds of years.

Ketones, also known as ketone bodies, are molecules produced by your liver when there is insufficient glucose in your body to provide the energy you require. These ketones, which are derived from fatty acids, supply your body with an alternate source of fuel, or energy, allowing you to perform the typical physiological tasks that keep you alive.

Ketones can aid increase cognitive function and mental performance by easily crossing the blood-brain barrier and providing a quick-acting source of energy to the brain. Ketones also give your body a consistent amount of physical energy. That's why many people feel more energized when they follow a ketogenic diet or use intermittent fasting.

There are three kinds of ketones:

AcAc (Acetoacetate)

Acetone

Beta-hydroxybutyrate (BHB)

Your liver always creates ketones, but the concentration of ketones in your blood is greatly influenced by your carbohydrate and protein consumption, as well as how frequently you eat. While high amounts of ketones can be deadly for people with type

1 diabetes, those with a perfectly functioning metabolism can handle them with ease. Any additional ketones that your body does not use as energy will be expelled when you breathe or pee.

Ketosis and Fasting

It usually takes approximately twelve hours of fasting to achieve the fat-burning state of ketosis, and things continue to pick up between hours sixteen and twenty-four. This is why many people advise fasting for sixteen hours. While this time range appears to work well for men, women usually perform better with shorter fasts of twelve to fourteen hours.

While you will begin to burn fat after around twelve hours, you will not achieve full nutritional ketosis. On average, this procedure takes two to four days if you eat less than 50 grams of carbohydrates per day. When the body produces ketones when fasting, it is usually insufficient to declare that you are in ketosis.

Advantages of fat adaptation

Being "fat-adapted" means that your body has adapted to using fat as its primary food source rather than carbs. This happens when you follow a low-carbohydrate, high-fat diet for an extended length of time (such as the ketogenic diet). Here are some of the advantages of fat adaptation:

Increased energy and endurance: Because fat is a more prolonged source of energy than carbs, fat-adapted people have more energy and endurance during activity.

Improved weight control: Fat-adapted people have a lower body fat percentage and more muscular mass, which can help with weight management.

Better blood sugar control: Because fat is used for fuel rather than glucose, fat-adapted people have more stable blood sugar levels, which can help prevent insulin resistance and type 2 diabetes.

Reduced inflammation: A high-carbohydrate diet can produce inflammation in the body, whereas a high-fat, low-carbohydrate diet can reduce inflammation and improve general health. Fat is a crucial component of brain tissue, and a fat-adapted diet can increase cognitive performance, memory, and focus.

Increased satiety: Because fat is more filling than carbs, fat-adapted people feel fuller after meals and are less prone to suffer cravings or hunger between meals.

How a high-carbohydrate diet can be harmful to one's health

Obesity risk increases: Eating too many carbs, particularly refined carbohydrates such as white bread, spaghetti, and sugary snacks, can lead to weight gain and obesity. Obesity is linked to several health problems, including type 2 diabetes, heart disease, and high blood pressure.

Insulin resistance: A high-carbohydrate diet can contribute to insulin resistance, which means the body becomes less efficient at using insulin to control blood sugar levels. Insulin resistance has been linked to an increased risk of type 2 diabetes, heart disease, and some malignancies.

Inflammation: Certain carbohydrate sources, such as refined grains and sweets, can promote inflammation in the body. Chronic inflammation has been related to a variety of health issues, including arthritis, heart disease, and cancer.

Risk of heart disease: A high carbohydrate diet, particularly refined carbohydrates, can raise the risk of heart disease. Excessive carbohydrate consumption can result in raised triglyceride levels in the blood, a kind of fat associated with an increased risk of heart disease.

Hormonal imbalances: A high-carbohydrate diet can cause

hormonal imbalances, particularly in middle-aged women.

High carbohydrate intake can cause insulin variations, which can impact the production of other hormones such as estrogen and progesterone. Hormonal imbalances can cause a variety of health problems, including irregular menstruation, weight gain, and mood swings. Overall, it is critical to maintain a well-balanced diet rich in a range of foods, including carbohydrates. Middle-aged women, on the other hand, should be cautious of their carbohydrate intake and focus on complex carbs such as whole grains, fruits, and vegetables, while minimizing their intake of processed carbohydrates and sugars.

Using fat for energy has various advantages:

1. Abundant Energy Source: Fat is a highly concentrated kind of energy. It has more than twice as many calories per gram as carbohydrates or protein. This means that by tapping into fat storage, the body can access a significant supply of energy.

2. Prolonged Sustained Energy: When you rely on fat for energy, it can give you a steady source of fuel. Unlike carbohydrates, which are quickly exhausted, fat stores are huge and can sustain energy production for longer periods. This is useful for endurance exercises or periods of sustained physical exertion.

3. Weight Control: Using fat for energy can help with weight control and fat removal. By causing an energy deficit, in which the body expends more energy than it consumes, fat stores can be mobilized and utilized, resulting in weight loss over time.

4. Increased Metabolic Flexibility: When the body gets more effective at using fat for energy, metabolic flexibility improves. This means that the body may more easily transition between using carbs and fats as fuel sources, adjusting to changing energy demands and dietary changes.

5. Lower Insulin Levels: Insulin levels tend to be lower when relying on fat for energy. Individuals with insulin resistance or diabetes may benefit from this since reduced insulin levels may aid improve blood sugar control.

Fat Adapted Diet: Sample meal plans and Recipes

A high-fat diet often involves increasing the quantity of healthy fats in your meals while decreasing carbohydrates. Here are some sample meal plans and dishes to get you started:

Breakfast:

Bulletproof Coffee: Combine 1 cup of hot coffee with 1 tablespoon of coconut oil and 1 tablespoon of grass-fed butter or ghee. Scrambled Eggs with Avocado: Scramble 2-3 eggs in 1 tablespoon of butter or ghee and serve with half an avocado.

Lunch:

Chicken Salad with Avocado: Combine cooked chicken breast, mayonnaise, diced celery, diced red onion, and diced avocado. Serve on a bed of lettuce. Greek Salad with Olive Oil Dressing: Toss lettuce, tomatoes, cucumbers, feta cheese, olives, and red onion with olive oil and lemon juice dressing.

Dinner:

Grilled meat with Garlic Butter: Season meat with salt and pepper and cook to the desired doneness. Serve with garlic butter made by combining softened butter and minced garlic. Baked Salmon with Lemon and Herbs: Season salmon filets with salt, pepper, lemon juice, and herbs such as thyme or rosemary. Bake for 10-12 minutes.

Snacks:

Cheese and nuts: Cheeses like cheddar or brie go well with nuts like almonds, cashews, and walnuts. Guacamole with Vegetable Sticks: Mash ripe avocados with lime juice and salt, then serve with celery or carrot sticks. Desserts: Chocolate Fat Bombs: Combine melted coconut oil, cocoa powder, and a sweetener like a stevia or erythritol in small moulds and freeze. Keto **Cheesecake:** Combine cream cheese, eggs, and almond extract in a mixing bowl and bake in the oven for a low-carb dessert

Adaptation to Fat and Exercise Regular exercise can help with fat adaption by improving the body's ability to burn fat when exercising. When you exercise, your body uses stored carbs as its primary source of energy. Regular endurance exercise, on the other hand, makes the body more efficient at using fat as fuel, which helps to save the body's limited glycogen stores in the muscles and liver. To enhance fat adaptation through exercise, it is necessary to engage in regular endurance training at a moderate level for an extended period, such as running, cycling, or swimming. This allows the body to progressively adapt to burning fat for fuel while still retaining glycogen reserves for high-intensity tasks.

It's also worth noting that fat adaption does not happen quickly and may require weeks or even months of persistent exercise. How exercise influences your body's energy use Exercise has several effects on your body's energy use. Here are some of the most important ways that exercise affects your energy levels:

Calorie burn increased: When you exercise, you burn more calories than when you are at rest. Calorie expenditure can originate from a variety of sources, including fat, carbs, and protein.

Improve metabolic rate: This means your body burns more calories even when you aren't exercising. This effect can linger for several hours after you finish working out.

Improved insulin sensitivity:

Regular exercise can increase your body's sensitivity to insulin, allowing your cells to use glucose (sugar) more efficiently. This can assist to stabilize your blood sugar levels and give you a consistent supply of energy throughout the day.

Enhances circulation :

which helps transport oxygen and nutrients to your muscles and other tissues. This can increase your overall energy levels and prevent weariness.

Increased endorphin production: Exercise can promote the creation of endorphins, which are natural "feel-good" compounds that can improve your mood and energy levels.

Overall, exercise can help you gain energy and enhance your health and well-being. Physical activity is an important aspect of living a healthy lifestyle since it can help you maintain a healthy weight, lower your risk of chronic diseases, and enhance your mental health.

Problems with Fat Adaptation

Common difficulties encountered when converting to a fat-adapted diet

For many people, switching to a fat-adapted diet can be a considerable lifestyle change. While there are numerous advantages to a fat-adapted diet, there are also some frequent obstacles that people may face throughout the adjustment. Here are a few examples: The keto flu: Some women may have flu-like symptoms when initially starting a fat-adapted diet, such as headaches, lethargy, and nausea. The "keto flu" is produced by the body adjusting to a new fuel source. These symptoms normally subside within a few days or weeks.

Cravings: When first converting to a fat-adapted diet, many women who are used to a high-carbohydrate diet may have carb cravings. This can be difficult to overcome, but it normally goes away as the body grows more acclimated to using fat as fuel.

Digestive problems: An abrupt increase in fat consumption can cause digestive problems such as bloating, constipation, and diarrhea. This could be because the body is adjusting to the new diet or because you are consuming too much fat too rapidly. Increasing fiber consumption and staying hydrated can assist with these symptoms.

Social challenges: eating a fat-adapted diet might be difficult in social settings where carb-heavy items are frequently served, such as restaurants and gatherings. Planning and packing your snacks, as well as doing some research on places that serve keto-friendly food, might be useful.

Monitoring macros: It's crucial to regularly monitor macronutrients if you want to keep up a fat-adapted diet. This can take time, and it can call for some learning and investigation.

How to Overcome These Obstacles

A high-fat diet can be difficult for some people to follow and maintain because it can lead to weight gain, an increased risk of heart disease, and other health problems. However, various ways can assist you in overcoming the difficulties of a high-fat diet: Choose healthy fats: Not all fats are the same. Avocados, almonds, seeds, olive oil, and fatty fish are all good sources of healthful fats. Concentrate on **whole foods:** Eating whole, unprocessed foods can assist you in avoiding the bad fats contained in many processed foods.

Watch your portion sizes: Even good fats can be heavy in calories, so keep track of your serving sizes and try to stay to them.

Include other macronutrients: Include meals high in protein and fiber in your diet to help balance your fat consumption and encourage satiety.

Stay physically active: Being physically active regularly can help you maintain a healthy weight and lower your risk of health problems associated with a high-fat diet.

Seek expert assistance: A trained dietician or a healthcare provider can assist you in developing a personalized plan that is best suited to your health objectives and dietary requirements. Remember that a high-fat diet is not for everyone, and it is critical to assess your personal health needs and goals before making any big dietary adjustments.

When should you seek expert assistance?

If you are considering or presently following a high-fat diet, it is critical to consult with a healthcare practitioner to evaluate if it is appropriate for you and to verify that you are fulfilling all of your nutritional needs. When following a high-fat diet, the following symptoms may suggest the need for expert assistance:

Unintentional weight loss or increase: Unintentional weight loss or gain may indicate that your high-fat diet is not balanced or healthy for your body.

Digestive difficulties: When following a high-fat diet, some people develop digestive disorders such as bloating, constipation, or diarrhea. If you suffer any of these symptoms, you must seek professional help.

Fatigue and weakness: Feeling weak or weary may indicate that you are not getting enough nutrients from your high-fat diet.

High cholesterol: A high-fat diet can raise your cholesterol levels, increasing your risk of heart disease. If you have excessive cholesterol or a family history of heart disease, you should seek professional advice before beginning a high-fat diet.

Diabetes: If you have diabetes or are at risk for diabetes, see a healthcare expert before beginning a high-fat diet, as it may not be appropriate for your situation

Conclusions

The recipes that fit in with the diet concepts have always been one of the essential keys to any successful diet or lifestyle change. I'm sure there are various strategies to stick to a healthy diet and lose weight. You don't want to get there by eating the same old meals over and over again.

We've arrived at this point, and I'm so delighted you've chosen to take the necessary steps on this journey. This book and its contents, I hope, will provide you with step-by-step actionable value for your journey towards healthful meal plans, as they always have.

More importantly, I hope that the book has boosted your confidence and strengthened your will to stick to the regimen.

Thank you for taking the time to read The Mid-Life Diet for Women. We hope that we have accomplished our major goal of providing you with all of the knowledge you could ever want on Intermittent Fasting, an Anti-inflammatory diet, Fuel Refocus, and how it impacts the female form. By the end of this guide, readers should have the knowledge and abilities necessary to not only begin their own unique Diet planning adventure but to do so with confidence in both their fasting schedule and themselves.

Remember that the goal of this guide is to provide information, practical measures to take, and guidance on how to grasp the foundations of dieting based on study and experience gathered and shared on the subject. It is not intended to be used as a medical reference or as the sole source of knowledge, especially for individuals who have pre-existing health conditions that may be affected by what and how much they consume daily. It is always a good idea, but also a necessary first step in attaining success through Dieting and Intermittent Fasting, to consult with a doctor before making any big changes to personal health plans, diets, or fitness routines.

We sincerely hope that now that you've learned the fundamentals of the middle age diet, what it is, and how it works, you'll be able to use it as a valuable support tool and regular lifestyle practices that will assist you in not only taking control of your health but also maintaining it throughout your life to become and enjoy being a healthier, happier version of yourself! Thank you for purchasing The Mid-Life Diet for Women, and best wishes on your particular health journey!

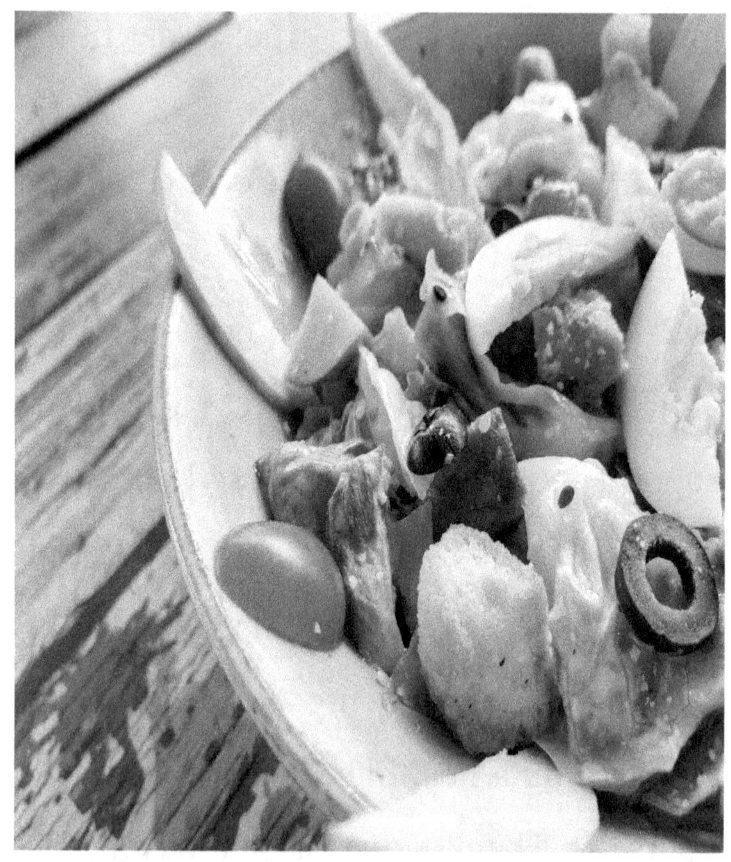

www.ingramcontent.com/pod-product-compliance
Lightning Source LLC
Chambersburg PA
CBHW070921260726

48661CB00003B/778